Hemodynamic Monitoring Made Easy

For Elsevier:
Senior Commissioning Editor: Ninette Premdas
Project Development Manager: Mairi McCubbin
Project Manager: David Fleming
Designer: Judith Wright
Illustrations Manager: Bruce Hogarth

Hemodynamic Monitoring Made Easy

Jayne A. D. Fawcett

BSc(Hons) MSc PGDipEd RGN ENB100/998

Team Leader, Intensive Therapy Unit,
St Georges Hospital,
London, UK

Forewords by

David Bennett

MB FRCP

Professor of Intensive Care Medicine,
St Georges Hospital,
London, UK

Barbara McLean

MN, RN, CCRN, CCNS, CCNP, FCCM

Nurse Intensivist,
Atlanta Medical Centre,
Atlanta Georgia, USA

ELSEVIER

EDINBURGH LONDON NEW YORK OXFORD PHILADELPHIA ST LOUIS SYDNEY TORONTO 2006

ELSEVIER

An imprint of Elsevier Limited

First published 2006

ISBN 0 7020 2781 2

British Library Cataloguing in Publication Data
A catalogue record for this book is available from the British Library

Library of Congress Cataloging in Publication Data
A catalog record for this book is available from the Library of Congress

Notice
Knowledge and best practice in this field are constantly changing. As new research and experience broaden our knowledge, changes in practice, treatment and drug therapy may become necessary or appropriate. Readers are advised to check the most current information provided (i) on procedures featured or (ii) by the manufacturer of each product to be administered, to verify the recommended dose or formula, the method and duration of administration, and contraindications. It is the responsibility of the practitioner, relying on their own experience and knowledge of the patient, to make diagnoses, to determine dosages and the best treatment for each individual patient, and to take all appropriate safety precautions. To the fullest extent of the law, neither the publisher nor the author assumes any liability for any injury and/or damage. *The Publisher*

Printed in China

Contents

Foreword

Nurses are playing an increasingly important role in the management of critically ill patients. They undertake a wide range of roles including setting up and running technologically advanced equipment such as hemodialsysers and modern ventilators.

One of the pivotal aspects in the managment of these patients is the monitoring and support of the cardiovascular system. Taking blood pressure and pulse rate is probably the commonest measurement that the nurse makes in most patients admitted to hospital. However, in the intensive care unit the nature of these measurements requires the nurse to have a much deeper understanding of the relationship between the measured variables and cardiovascular function. Not only do these variables have to be measured accurately but the results have to be interpreted and adjustments made to the treatment the patient is usually receiving. This places a very considerable burden of responsibility on the nurse.

Over the years this burden has increased considerably. New technologies are constantly being introduced and choices have to be made as to which should be used. Nurses' views are important because it is nurses who are likely to be the main users of the new devices. Thus they must develop an intimate understanding of the technology which then has to be introduced into the high pressure environment of the intensive care unit. Furthermore, junior members of staff will have to be taught how to use this new equipment.

Similar issues arise with young physicians in training who

will often spend only a short time in the intensive care unit. Their understanding of the body's circulation is often limited and rarely are they aware of the problems involved in monitoring it.

It is therefore particularly pleasing and appropriate that a senior member of nursing staff on the intensive care unit at St George's has single-handedly written a book which covers all these issues in considerable detail. It is appropriate because the intensive care unit at St George's has had a long-standing interest in the circulation with particular emphasis on how its manipulation improves outcome in high-risk surgical patients.

Indeed it was through this interest that we first got to know Jayne Fawcett as she was one of the principal authors of a very important paper showing how increasing cardiac output reduces mortality and length of hospital stay in patients having major surgery. After joining us she again made a major contribution in another paper addressing the same issues.

She has therefore acquired an in-depth knowledge of the circulation and how it can be monitored and manipulated. Her book is wide-ranging and gives detailed information in a concise and readable form. It should become standard reading for all intensive care nurses and junior doctors who have any interest in expanding their usually limited knowledge of the circulation.

London, 2005   David Bennett

Foreword

For over thirty years we have been monitoring the blood flow dynamics of our intensive care patients with right heart (pulmonary artery) catheters. In our attempts to diagnose, intervene and improve outcomes we progressed rapidly with data, despite the paucity of understanding of the information measured. Since 1995, evidence has confirmed the abundance of misconception and misdiagnosis of patients based on poorly delineated data. Since the landmark studies of Conner and Iberti, as well as the guidelines introduced by the Society of Critical Care Medicine, the use of the pulmonary artery catheter has been the object of discussion and debate, with stakeholders on both sides. I, for one, firmly believe that the value of the right heart catheter is as essential to the management of specific patients as ventilators are to the control of respiration. Having said that, I must admit that even today, a great deal of my time is spent in educating nurses, residents and others in the basic components of waveform analysis and right and left heart disconnect in extraordinary critical illness.

About three years ago, I had the pleasure of meeting Jayne Fawcett at the European Society of Critical Care medicine annual meeting in Barcelona, Spain. I was immediately in awe of the breadth and depth of her knowledge and influence in the European community, particularly with regard to hemodynamic monitoring and severe shock states.

As we all search for endpoints of value in the resuscitation and management of critical patients, Ms Fawcett was evolving the clinical practice of evaluation to a new level. Working with many physician and nurse colleagues, Ms

Fawcett became a renowned expert in the utilization of oesophageal Doppler catheters and the development of nurse-driven guidelines for hemodynamic management. She further evolved the state of the art of left heart measurements of stroke volume variability and systolic pressure variation with her dedicated and insightful work with pulse contour technology, in particular Lithium Derived cardiac output.

The sentinel work of hemodynamic experts like Elaine Dailey and Dr Tom Ahrens introduced the basic understanding of hemodynamic concepts. Others followed with more explicit methods for assuring waveform analysis, mixed and central venous oxygenation, incorporating the endpoint of cellular dynamics as we began to unfold the mysteries of shock states, in particular severe sepsis. In the last ten years, the value and diagnostic validity of the pulmonary catheter has spurred multiple debates internationally. The works of Bennett, Rhinehart, Fawcett, Payen, Rivers, and Pinsky, among many others, has provided new paths for exploration of both right and left heart dynamics and may add further controversy as well as elucidation.

Fawcett's intelligent, simple, and comprehensive guide not only reviews the basic concepts of traditional hemodynamic monitoring, but takes the practitioner into complete and relevant discussions of the multitude of diagnostic advances applied at the bedside. Jayne Fawcett's *Hemodynamic Monitoring Made Easy* bursts with information in a user-friendly, profoundly engaging, straightforward manner. Suitable for novice, expert, nurse and physician, this book answers a long-awaited deficit. Up-to-date information based on the known structures of pressure vs volume, waveforms, gases and tissue issues. Beyond any other guide currently available, Fawcett has progressed the art of hemodynamic interpretation to the ICU of today.

Enjoy!

Atlanta Georgia, 2005   Barbara McLean

Preface

This book has been written following many years of clinical experience spent managing critically ill patients' hemodynamic status, using a range of techniques and technologies, in the clinical setting, in a lecturer's role and as part of clinical research. The book does not intend to provide the reader with practical advice on how to use these technologies, for example, how to switch the equipment on! Rather, the intention is to help the reader understand the underlying technical, physical and mechanical principles that these technologies are based upon. This knowledge, together with a sound understanding of anatomy and physiology, will then allow the reader to apply these principles to any technology in order to help them solve problems and troubleshoot when dealing with everyday critical care technology used to generate hemodynamic data.

This book focuses on the link between the basic and complex physiological principles that help us to understand hemodynamic monitoring. In addition, it explains the sources and nature of the electrical, chemical and mechanical events that occur with each heartbeat and how to interpret these signals on the monitor. Only then can nurses make informed decisions about what is happening to a patient's hemodynamic status.

Hemodynamic monitoring isn't just about inserting lines and connecting the patient to a monitoring system. The quality of the information you then obtain is very dependent upon the attention to detail of the nurse at the bedside. If the nurse is unaware or unable to obtain accurate data you might as well write down the data from the patient in the next bed for all the use it will be. Obtaining this quality of information depends on several factors. First, the equipment at the bedside and the nurse's ability to recognize a technical, mechanical or electrical problem. Second, to have not only an understanding of normal physiology and the different ways, not only to collect, but also to interpret the information obtained from chemical, mechanical and electrical signals generated. An important point is being able to look at all the data presented and be able to make the physiological link between them. This is the only way that the information can be of any use clinically.

Even the most-experienced intensive care nurse can find that a gap in knowledge exists; fairly fundamental aspects can somehow be missed early on in the nurse's intensive care career. Often this is because, when first starting in intensive care, both nurses and doctors can be overwhelmed by the equipment, treatment and environment, so small, but important details can be missed. Before you know it, you will have been in intensive care for some time before a student or junior colleague asks a question you cannot answer. That has happened to me more times than I care to remember. Because of this, I think this book will be useful to both new intensive care nurses and those with much more experience, to update themselves on the new technologies available and fill any gaps in knowledge they may have. Furthermore, I hope that those teaching critical care will find it a useful source of information.

It is important to foster an awareness of current evidence-based thinking in relation to the hemodynamic monitoring and management of patients. In order to facilitate this, the book begins with a section on cardiovascular physiology, as a reminder of the importance of understanding how the structure of the cardiovascular system is linked to its function, particularly in relation to the important parameters we monitor, measure and use to guide therapies. These parameters are covered in detail, in a way that makes the sometimes complex subject of hemodynamic monitoring 'easy'. To be consistent with this approach, the book uses abbreviations sparingly to avoid confusion due to less-familiar terms, particularly when trying to get to grips with new or complex concepts. An extensive glossary is included at the end.

The book aims to enable the reader to:
- appreciate the importance of clinical observations in the cardiovascular assessment of patients, particularly before monitoring has been established
- know how to obtain accurate data from cardiovascular monitors
- understand the difference between the information gained from non-invasive and invasive equipment
- understand and be able to check the accuracy of monitors and transduced waveforms
- identify each waveform component of an arterial/central venous/pulmonary artery (and wedge) pressure/bioimpedence and oesophageal Doppler; pulse/systolic and stroke volume variations
- be able to make the link of each to the electrical, chemical and mechanical events and signals from the cardiovascular and respiratory systems
- understand the uses and limitations of the arterial blood, central venous blood and pulmonary artery blood pressures, and pulmonary artery wedge pressures
- understand cardiac output and its components, and the delivery, consumption and extraction of oxygen as indicators of adequate hydration and tissue perfusion
- understand the interactions that take place between the heart and lungs, their effect on stroke volume throughout the respiratory cycle and how they may be used to guide fluid therapy in mechanically ventilated patients

- know what systolic pressure variation, pulse pressure variation, stroke volume variation, extravascular lung water and interthoracic blood volume are, and their clinical use
- understand why less-invasive methods of estimating cardiac output are increasingly being used
- be able to compare/contrast and understand the strengths and weaknesses of the Thermodilution (Pulmonary artery catheter), Fick (NICO), Transthoracic Bioimpedence (Bio Z), Doppler Ultrasonography (Cardiac Q), Indicator dilution (LiDCO) and Transpulmonary thermo-dilution (PiCCO) used to estimate cardiac output
- understand what Optimization/Goal-directed therapy is and the benefits to patients, particularly when it is nurse-led.

Some very good books on hemodynamic monitoring are available, however, none of them cover all of the technologies currently available to measure cardiac output less invasively, in particular pulse contour analysis. This book is unique in that respect. All technologies currently available are considered, with the emphasis on the underlying principles rather than the monitors themselves.

London, 2005   Jayne A. D. Fawcett

Acknowledgements

This book was written following many years of questioning what hemodynamic monitoring was about and how it really influenced what happened to the patients in my care. During this journey there have been many individuals who have influenced not only my thinking but also how I have presented this book. I would like to thank Deborah Dawson and Annie Palmer and all the nursing and medical staff in the general intensive care unit at St Georges Hospital, London, who have given much of their time on many occasions to listen to my anxieties, but have also contributed to and fed my ideas. My special thanks must go to Kashif Ikram, without whom I would not have had the confidence to propose or finish this book. Finally, I would very much like to thank my beautiful daughter, Julie. Her infinite support and encouragement has kept me grounded during some very stressful times and I will always be grateful and proud of her for that.

Introduction and overview

It is generally accepted that hemodynamic monitoring is an essential component in the overall assessment of the critically ill patient. In addition, the accurate measurement and determination of a patient's cardiac function is a necessary means of assessing the response to therapeutic interventions. The interpretation of this information is required in order to make many decisions both rapidly and efficiently. To do this, a sound physiological and pathophysiological knowledge base is required. Numbers by themselves are of no use without the ability to interpret what they mean. A single parameter is unlikely to provide all the information needed to make sound clinical decisions about a patient's management. What is important is to know how a single piece of information may fit into the overall picture.

Ultimately, the aim of hemodynamic monitoring is to assess the adequacy of tissue perfusion with accuracy and precision. Having said that, we still know very little about patient monitoring and no trial exists that proves that the monitoring of vital signs, in itself, improves outcome. There is a great deal of data out there but it is often confusing. What seems to be important is the ability to recognize when the body's normal homeostatic mechanisms have been triggered, and also what we measure as much as how we measure it, especially in relation to the risks to the patient. After all, monitoring, itself, is not therapy! In the future, I believe that global hemodynamic monitoring will be enhanced by monitoring regional circulations and biochemical markers, and by further exploring the role of the mitochondria in ways that are minimally invasive. Most of these developments are already being addressed.

The body is able to give us many important signals and clues as to whether it is in a homeostatic state or not. Having said that, there are individual variations. For example, young people, particularly children, can compensate physiologically for quite catastrophic events that are occurring internally, until the body reaches the point at which it is no longer able to maintain a homeostatic state. There are many sources of signals in the body that can also potentially provide us with some insight into the body's physical qualities, such as flow, volume, pressure, voltage, charge, sound, absorption and elasticity (resistance). These signals can be spontaneous bioelectrical signals, such as the modulation of energy (pulse oximetry) and the electrocardiogram (ECG), or bioelectrical, as in voltage- and chemically gated channels, pumps and ionic imbalances, as in the action potential. Shearing forces produce turbulence and this can be heard as sounds. Auscultation also provides us with heart, respiratory and circulatory sounds.

Waveforms do provide details that can, with diagnoses, confirm digital values, or warn when these values should be questioned. Flushing/patients' movement and electrical interference (artifacts) can distort both waveforms and digital values, giving inaccurate values. However, as already mentioned, in order to interpret waveforms, an appreciation of cardiac and circulatory anatomy and physiology is essential. The assessment and adequacy of cardiac preload is fundamental in the management of the critically ill patient. Inadequate preload may lead to compromised tissue perfusion and multiorgan failure, whereas excessive fluid loading may result in the development of pulmonary oedema and worsening respiratory function, which may contribute to both morbidity and mortality.

The management of critically ill patients is based on knowledge of fundamental physiological variables. Monitoring techniques of the hemodynamic status of these patients has developed considerably from the non-invasive monitoring of a single parameter to more invasive monitoring of multiple parameters. This can lead to a far more comprehensive picture and analysis, allowing those looking after the patient to anticipate events and provide more efficient treatment. In reality, very few of our monitors are truly specific. The pulse oximeter may indicate a drop in arterial saturation; however, this could be due to low inspired oxygen, a decrease in cardiac output, a fall in the temperature of the extremity, an injection of dye, or nail polish. The ECG can note tachycardia but this may be due to pain, inadequate anesthesia, hypovolemia, or a medication that has just been injected. Likewise, a fall in the heart rate can have as many causes. The blood pressure might be reduced with hypovolemia, tachycardia or bradycardia, decrease in venous return or a relative overdose of an anesthetic. The pulmonary capillary wedge pressure (PCWP) might decrease with a fall in volume or because the cardiac output has increased. An increased PCWP could indicate a change in volume status or impending cardiac failure. Urine output may depend on volume status, previous diuretic therapy, cardiac output or blood pressure. None of these are really specific. Clinicians use their experience and assessment of all the variables before deciding on the cause of an alteration in their patient's condition. Only then can the appropriate response be determined and carried out.

There is not one piece of electronic equipment that can replace knowledgeable, trained critical care staff who are capable of intervening on behalf of the patient. Modern technology is of little value unless it is continuous, works properly, and generates information that can be interpreted correctly and applied appropriately. The individual who has responsibility for doing these things must be capable in order to ensure safe care and management of the patient.

Understanding the basis of hemodynamic monitoring

1 The cardiovascular system

Main objectives

- Outline the location, size and position of the heart in the thoracic cavity.
- Identify the layers, heart chambers and sounds of the heart, and describe their function.
- Identify the valves and discuss the functions of each.
- Trace blood flow through the heart, and compare the functions of the heart chambers on the right and left sides.
- Describe the blood supply to the heart and the effects of the autonomic nervous system on heart function.
- List the anatomical components of the heart's conduction system.
- Identify the electrical events associated with the normal electrocardiogram and explain the mechanical events of the cardiac cycle.

Overview of the cardiovascular system

Before we can begin to unfold the complexities of hemodynamic monitoring, both simple and basic, it makes sense to review how the structure and function of the cardiovascular system result in signals that we can use to guide therapy in the critically ill patient. Having said that, the whole of this chapter refers to how the cardiovascular system is structured and should function in health. Later chapters will demonstrate how, in critical illness, patients' cardiovascular systems are rarely structured or function normally, and this affects our interpretation of the body signals we monitor and, therefore, our management of the patient.

Ultimately, the cardiovascular system aims to provide sufficient oxygen to every tissue in the body so that the mitochondria (the power house of the cell) can produce energy (adenosine triphosphate; ATP) at a rate that meets the ever-changing demands of the body, both in health and in critical illness (Brooker 1993).

In 1628, the English physician, William Harvey, demonstrated that blood flows in one direction throughout the blood vessels and, therefore, discovered that blood does, in fact, circulate (the circulatory system). Before this, it had been believed that blood flowed in and out of the heart through the same vessels. Through dissections conducted by anatomists, it became clear that the large vessels that were attached to the heart branched off into smaller and smaller vessels, finally ending up at major organs. Smaller microscopic vessels that connected to these branches, and any loops or circuits they formed could not be identified (microscopes had not been invented at this point). The anatomical link between arteries, veins and capillaries was not made until later in the 17th century, when Marcello

Malpighi, an Italian physiologist, observed capillaries through a microscope.

We now know that blood flows through a network of blood vessels that extend between the heart and the peripheral tissues (Figure 1.1). These blood vessels can be subdivided into the pulmonary circuit, which carries blood to and from the gas exchange surfaces of the lungs, and the systemic circuit, which transports blood to and from the rest of the body. Each circuit begins and ends at the heart, and blood travels through these circuits in sequence. Arteries carry blood away from the heart (except in the case of the pulmonary artery) and veins carry blood towards the heart (except in the case of the pulmonary veins). The capillaries are small, thin-walled vessels between the smallest arteries and veins. The thin walls of capillaries permit the exchange of nutrients, dissolved gases and waste products between the blood and the tissues surrounding it (Rutishauser 1997, Marieb 2001, 2003).

Despite the hearts considerable workload, it is small, only being the size of a clenched fist. It contains four muscular chambers. The right atrium receives blood from the systemic circuit (superior and inferior vena cava) and passes it to the right ventricle. The right ventricle pumps blood into the pulmonary circuit (pulmonary artery). The left atrium collects blood from the pulmonary circuit (pulmonary vein) and empties it into the left ventricle. Contraction of the left ventricle then ejects blood into the systemic circuit (aorta). When the heart beats, the atria contract first, then the ventricles contract. The two ventricles contract at the same time and eject equal volumes of blood into the pulmonary and systemic circuits (Soloman & Davies 1996, Seeley 2000). Blood is carried away from the heart by arteries and returned by way of veins. Capillaries interconnect the smallest arteries (arterioles) and the smallest veins (venules), and exchange nutrients, dissolved gases and

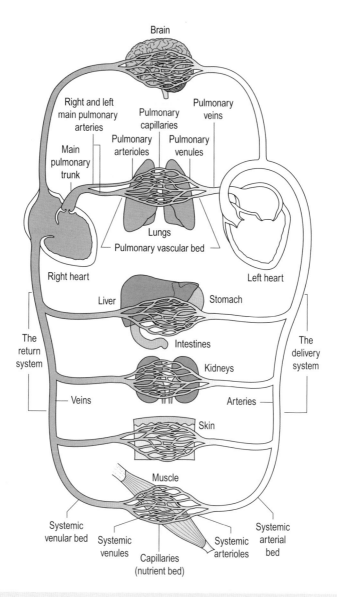

Fig 1.1 Cardiovascular circuit. (Reproduced with permission from Darovic 2002).

waste products between the blood and the surrounding tissues (Thibodeau & Patton 2003).

The anatomy of blood vessels

In health, the cardiovascular system is a closed circuit, with blood being contained within arteries, arterioles (smaller arteries), capillaries, venules (smaller veins), veins and the heart. Any leakage of fluid that occurs from the capillaries is returned to the cardiovascular circuit via the lymphatic system (Thibodeau & Patton 2003).

The walls of both arteries and veins have the same three distinct layers. They have an external tunica externa, a middle tunica media and an innermost tunica interna (this layer is smooth to prevent turbulent blood flow). These layers not only give strength to the vessels, but also their muscular and elastic properties allow the diameter of the vessels to be modified according to the demand of the body for changes in pressure or volume of blood (Marieb 2003). The walls of arteries and veins differ; this is to allow for the conditions in which they have to function. Arteries are much thicker than veins (which helps them to retain their shape under pressure) and contain more smooth muscle and elastic fibers. This is because they have to absorb pressure coming from the ventricle during contraction (the highest pressure being in the aorta). The internal lumen of an artery is smaller than a vein because of its muscular layer. The walls of veins are also thinner. This is because the pressure in them is not as great as that in the arteries and, therefore, they do not need to have such a thick muscular layer (Saladin 1997, Marieb 2003). Although thinner, the internal diameter of veins is much greater. Limb veins contain valves to assist the return of blood from the peripheral circulation back to the heart. These valves also prevent backflow of blood towards the

Quiz 1.1

1. *Do you know how the structure of an artery differs from that of a vein and why this is?*

2. *Can you identify the three layers of blood vessels?*

capillaries. Capillaries are the only blood vessels to allow the exchange of fluids between the blood and surrounding tissues. The flow of blood through capillaries is slow and their walls are thin. This allows diffusion to occur quickly and exchange to be efficient. The blood volume content of each of these blood vessels is also different, with the largest proportion of blood being contained within the venous system (Marieb 2003, Thibodeau & Patton 2003).

Blood cannot be compressed. This is because it is a liquid. Any force against a liquid creates hydrostatic pressure. If a pressure gradient exists, hydrostatic pressure will push liquid from an area of higher pressure to an area of lower pressure. In the systemic circulation, the pressure gradient is the circulatory pressure. This is the pressure difference that exists between the aorta and the right atrium. It is the existence of this pressure that forces blood through the arterioles and into the capillaries (Seeley 2000, Tortora & Grabowski 2003). This pressure has three components – blood pressure (force exerted against vessel walls), capillary hydrostatic pressure (fluid pressure in capillaries), and venous pressure (pressure in the venous system).

Anatomy of the heart and valves

Many of the structural features of the heart can be seen when it is cut open. This organ is hollow and a partition (septum) divides it into right and left sides (Figure 1.2).

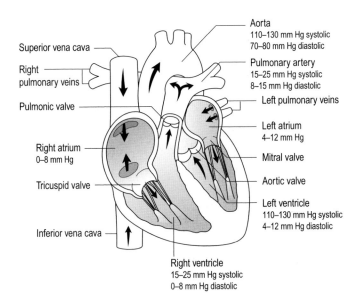

Superior vena cava

Right pulmonary veins

Pulmonic valve

Right atrium
0–8 mm Hg

Tricuspid valve

Inferior vena cava

Aorta
110–130 mm Hg systolic
70–80 mm Hg diastolic

Pulmonary artery
15–25 mm Hg systolic
8–15 mm Hg diastolic

Left pulmonary veins

Left atrium
4–12 mm Hg

Mitral valve

Aortic valve

Left ventricle
110–130 mm Hg systolic
4–12 mm Hg diastolic

Right ventricle
15–25 mm Hg systolic
0–8 mm Hg diastolic

Fig 1.2 The flow of blood through the normal heart. (Reproduced with permission from Darovic 2002).

The heart wall itself comprises of three distinct layers (Figure 1.3). Each chamber is lined by a thin layer of very smooth muscle tissue, called endothelium (or the endo-cardium). The heart is surrounded by a pericardial cavity. The heart's outer covering is the pericardium (parietal and visceral layers with a small space in between containing pericardial fluid). The pericardial sac stabilizes the position of the heart and associated vessels within the mediasternum (Seeley 2000). The myocardium is the muscular wall of the heart (containing blood vessels and nerves) and forms both the atria and the ventricles. The atria are smaller than the ventricles, and their walls are thinner and less muscular. The interatrial septum separates the atria, while the much thicker interventricular septum separates the ventricles (Thibodeau & Patton 2003).

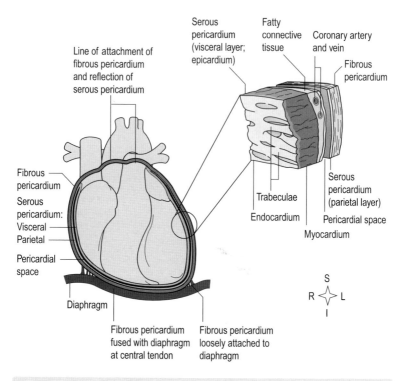

Fig 1.3 Wall of the heart. (Reproduced with permission from Thibodeau & Patton 2003).

The valves of the heart maximize the pumping action of the heart (two atrioventricular valves – the tricuspid and mitral; two semilunar valves – the pulmonary and aortic). These valves are folds of fibrous tissue. The chordae tendineae and papillary muscles play an important role by stopping the cusps of the valves from swinging in the wrong direction. These symmetrical cusps support one another like tripod legs (Marieb 2003).

The two atrioventricular valves prevent the backflow of blood into the atria when the ventricles contract. The pulmonary valve prevents blood from flowing back into the

Quiz 1.2

1. The heart wall comprises three layers. Can you identify them and state the function of each?

2. Can you identify the heart valves and discuss their function in relation to the cardiac cycle?

Quiz 1.3

1. Can you trace the flow of blood through the heart, identifying the chambers and valves?

2. Can you compare the function of the right side of the heart with that of the left?

right ventricle. The aortic valve prevents blood from flowing back into the left ventricle (Rutishauser 1997, Seeley 2000, Thibodeau & Patton 2003).

The supply of blood to the heart

The supply of blood to the heart is by way of the coronary circulation. The coronary circulation comprises of an extensive network of blood vessels, distributing blood to and from the heart itself. The heart works continuously, and cardiac muscle cells require reliable supplies of oxygen and nutrients (Marieb 2003). Myocardial blood supply comes from the right and left coronary arteries, which run over the surface of the heart, giving branches to the endocardium (the inner layer of the myocardium). Venous drainage is mostly via the coronary sinus into the right atrium. Having said that, a small proportion of blood flows directly into the ventricles, delivering unoxygenated blood to the systemic circulation (Marieb 2003). Oxygen extraction by the tissues is dependent on consumption and delivery. Myocardial oxygen consumption is higher than that in skeletal muscle: 75% of arterial oxygen is extracted by the myocardium compared to 25% by skeletal muscle (Thibodeau & Patton 2003). This means that any increased myocardial metabolic demand must be matched by an increase in coronary blood flow. This is a local response, which results in changes in the tone of the coronary arteries, with only a small amount of input from the autonomic nervous system (Marieb 2003, Thibodeau & Patton 2003).

Autoregulation

Regulation of blood flow within an organ is controlled by vasoconstrictors and vasodilators. These substances are released by the tissues surrounding blood vessels and by an internal mechanism within the vascular smooth muscle. This is local regulation. In addition, there are several external mechanisms that regulate the diameter of blood vessels by acting upon the vessels themselves. They are activated in response to the needs of the body for changes in pressure, volume and flow. One of these mechanisms is brought about by the existence of an autonomic nerve supply to blood vessels (Marieb 2003). Under normal conditions, this sympathetic vascular tone causes both resistance and venous capacitance vessels to be partially constricted. Circulating vasoactive hormones, such as angiotensin II, epinephrine, norepinephrine, vasopressin (antidiuretic hormone; ADH), atrionatriuretic peptide (ANP) and endothelin, represent a second external mechanism that alters the resistance of blood vessels (Seeley 2000, Tortora & Grabowski 2003).

The resistance to blood flow within the vascular system is determined by:

Quiz 1.4

1. *What is the resistance to blood flow determined by?*
2. *Which is the most important and why?*
3. *How is the flow of blood regulated within an organ?*
4. *Can you outline the external mechanisms that regulate blood vessel diameter?*

- the size of the individual blood vessels (both length and diameter);
- the organization of the vascular network (arrangements);
- the properties of blood (viscosity, laminar versus turbulent flow); and
- the external mechanical forces affecting the vasculature.

The most important of these factors for regulating blood flow to organs and blood pressure are changes in the diameter of blood vessels (Saladin 1997). The ability to change the diameter of arterioles in particular allows the body to adjust flow to tissues according to the changing metabolic demand. If an organ needs to alter its blood flow, the cells surrounding these blood vessels release vasoactive substances, which can either constrict or dilate the resistance vessels. In organs such as the heart and skeletal muscles, it is the contraction and relaxation itself that creates compressive forces, which can decrease vessel diameter and increase resistance to flow (Marieb 2003, Thibodeau & Patton 2003).

Nerve supply to the heart

The heart depends on a nerve supply from the brain (autonomic nervous system) that is able to respond automatically to changes in the demands of the body for oxygen. It does this by controlling and altering (regulating) both the rate and force of each cardiac contraction, after having received and interpreted messages from the many types of receptors that are located throughout the body. Both the sympathetic (stimulatory – speeds up) and parasympathetic (inhibitory – slows down) divisions of the autonomic nervous system supply the heart via the cardiac plexus (Marieb 2003, Thibodeau & Patton 2003).

Sympathetic nerve endings can be found in the muscle of the atria and ventricles, sinoatrial node and atrioventricular junction. Parasympathetic nerve endings occur mainly in atrial muscle, the sinoatrial node (pacemaker) and the atrioventricular junction (Seeley 2000). The target organs of the sympathetic nervous system contain receptors for norepinepherine and epinephrine (Thibodeau & Patton 2003). Sympathetic stimulation has a positive inotropic effect, causing the release of norepinephrine and the secretion of epinephrine and norepinephrine by the adrenal medulla. In addition to their effects on heart rate, these hormones (neurotransmitters) stimulate cardiac muscle metabolism, and increase the force and degree of contraction by stimulating alpha and beta receptors in the cell membranes of cardiac muscle (Thibodeau & Patton 2003). The release of these hormones results in the ventricles contracting more forcefully, increasing the ejection fraction and decreasing end systolic volume (Thibodeau & Patton 2003).

Parasympathetic stimulation supplies the heart via the vagus nerve. Parasympathetic stimulation has a negative inotropic effect, and its effects are limited to the sinoatrial node and the atrioventricular junction. The primary effect of acetylcholine (the hormone involved) is at the surface of the membrane, where it produces hyperpolarization (augmentation of the action potential) and inhibition (Marieb 2003). The result is a decrease in heart rate through its effects

Quiz 1.5

1. Can you describe the supply of blood to and from the heart?

2. Do you know how the heart is supplied with nerves and from which part of the nervous system?

3. Do you know which neurotransmitters are involved in the autonomic nervous system control of the heart?

on the sinoatrial and atrioventricular nodes. The force and rate of cardiac contractions is also reduced. There is little or no parasympathetic supply to the ventricles; therefore, the greatest changes are seen in the atria. Having said that, under strong parasympathetic stimulation or after the administration of drugs that mimic the actions of acetylcholine, the ventricles contract less forcefully, the ejection fraction decreases and the end-systolic volume increases (Seeley 2000, Marieb 2003, Thibodeau & Patton 2003).

The conduction system

The heart rate is controlled by autonomic nerve signals. However, the heart has its own built-in conduction system for coordinating contractions during the cardiac cycle (Thibodeau & Patton 2003). All the cardiac muscle fibers in each region of the heart are linked together electrically by intercalated disks, which combine to form a single unit that is capable of conducting an impulse through the entire wall of the heart without stopping. This is an important point. The walls of both the atria and ventricles will contract at about the same time because of this (Marieb 2003).

In the walls of the heart, four structures are embedded. These structures, the sinoatrial node, the atrioventricular

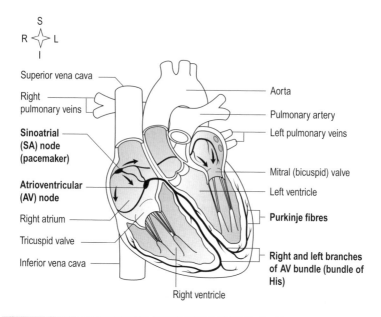

S
R ⟨⟩ L
I

Superior vena cava

Right pulmonary veins

Sinoatrial (SA) node (pacemaker)

Atrioventricular (AV) node

Right atrium

Tricuspid valve

Inferior vena cava

Aorta

Pulmonary artery

Left pulmonary veins

Mitral (bicuspid) valve

Left ventricle

Purkinje fibres

Right and left branches of AV bundle (bundle of His)

Right ventricle

Fig 1.4 Conduction system of the heart. (Reproduced with permission from Thibodeau & Patton 2003).

junction, the bundle of His and Purkinje fibers, are all specialized to generate strong impulses and to conduct them rapidly to regions of the heart wall to make sure atrial and ventricular contraction is achieved efficiently (Figure 1.4). A sequence of changes in the membrane of all cardiac muscle cells occurs to bring about the contraction (Marieb 2003, Seeley 2000).

The heartbeat (chemical events)

In a single heartbeat, the entire heart, atria and ventricles contract in a coordinated manner so that blood flows in the right direction at the right time. Each time the heart beats, two types of cardiac muscle cells must contract in sequence

Quiz 1.6

1. *Can you identify the two types of cardiac muscle cell?*
2. *Can you describe the function of each?*
3. *Do you know how the heart rate is controlled?*
4. *Can you list the components of the conducting system of the heart?*

(Thibodeau & Patton 2003). Contractile cells produce the powerful contraction that propels blood. Specialized muscle cells of the conducting system control and coordinate the activities of those contractile cells. Each complete heartbeat is called a 'cardiac cycle' and, in simple terms, includes the contraction (systole) and relaxation (diastole) of the atria and ventricles. Each cycle takes about 0.8 seconds to complete, if the heart rate is about 72 beats/minute. The electrical pacemaker (sinoatrial node) and conduction system sets the normal rhythm of the heart and coordinates its contraction (Marieb 2003). Cardiac muscle cells can contract rhythmically by themselves; however, they must be coordinated by electrical impulses in order for the heart to pump effectively. This process (an action potential) proceeds in the following three sequential steps.

Rapid depolarization (voltage-gated, fast Na^+ channels open)

Contractile cardiac muscle fibers have a resting potential of $-90\,mV$ (Seeley 2000). When brought to threshold by excitation in neighboring fibers, voltage-gated, fast sodium (Na^+) channels open very rapidly. Sodium ions rush into the cells (because of the concentration of Na^+ that exists inside and outside the cells), producing a rapid depolarization (change in electrical charge).

Plateau (voltage-gated, slow Ca^{2+} channels open)

Voltage-gated, slow calcium (Ca^{2+}) channels open in the plasma membrane (sarcolemma) and the membrane of the sarcoplasmic reticulum. As a result, calcium diffuses into the cytoplasm from the extracellular fluid and sarcoplasmic reticulum (again because of the concentration of Ca^{2+} that exists inside and outside the cells). The combined build-up of sodium and calcium ions in the cytoplasm maintains depolarization for about 250 ms (Marieb 2003; Thibodeau & Patton 2003)

Repolarization (voltage-gated, K^+ channels open)

During repolarization, potassium (K^+) channels open and potassium ions diffuse out of the cell into the extracellular fluid (again because of the concentration of K^+ that exists inside and outside the cells). At the same time, the Na^+ and Ca^{2+} channels are closing. The resting membrane potential of -90 mV is restored and the muscle fiber relaxes (Thibodeau & Patton 2003).

The refractory period of cardiac muscle prevents the heart from seizing up. It refers to the period of time when a muscle or nerve cell is unresponsive to stimulation. There are two refractory periods: absolute and relative. During the

---

Quiz 1.7

1. *Can you list the sequential steps of an action potential that occur at the cellular level?*

2. *Can you identify the important electrolytes involved in cardiac conduction?*

> ### TERMINOLOGY BOX 1.1
>
> **PR interval** – 0.12–0.20 s
>
> **QRS duration** – 0.08–0.12 s
>
> **QT interval** – 0.25–0.45 s

absolute refractory period, the cells remain unresponsive to any stimulus, regardless of its strength. During the relative refractory period, if the impulse is strong enough, a further action potential could be generated (Seeley 2000, Thibodeau & Patton 2003).

The cardiac cycle (mechanical events)

The proper functioning of the cardiac conduction system, together with the coordination of valve opening and closing in each region of the heart, is critical for efficient pumping of the blood (Figure 1.5). Each phase of the cardiac cycle is described in detail below.

During atrial systole (contraction), the atrioventricular valves are open and the semilunar valves are closed. The sinoatrial node, picked up on the surface as the P-wave of the electrocardiogram (ECG) – which you will remember represents electrical depolarization of the atria, initiates contraction of the atria. As the atria contract, the pressure within them increases so that a pressure gradient is generated across the open atrioventricular valves, causing a rapid flow of blood into the ventricles. Backflow from the atria into the vena cava is prevented by force of venous return and by the wave of contraction causing a milking effect throughout the atria (Marieb 2003, Thibodeau & Patton 2003). Ordinarily, contraction of the atria only accounts for

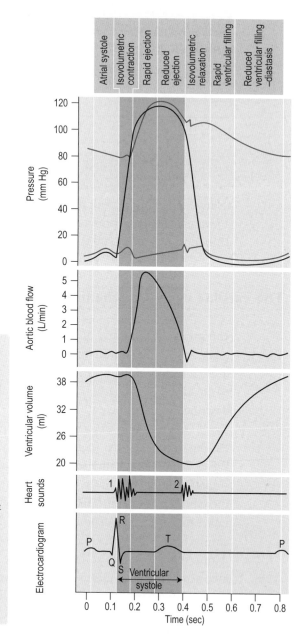

Fig 1.5 Chart of heart function. It comprises several diagrams: cardiac pumping cycle, blood pressure, flow and volume, the electrocardiogram and heart sounds. It is designed to give you a feel for all the different mechanical, electrical and chemical events that occur during one heartbeat, and is worth revisiting as you work through the book. (Reproduced with permission from Thibodeau & Patton 2003).

about 10% of left ventricular filling when a person is at rest (Thibodeau & Patton 2003). This is because most of the ventricular filling occurs before the atria contract and, therefore, is passive. Having said that, if the heart rate is very high (e.g. while exercising), contraction of the atria may account for as much as 40% of ventricular filling. The contribution of the atria to ventricular filling does vary depending on the duration of ventricular diastole (relaxation), and directly with contractility of the atria (Seeley 2000).

After contraction of the atria is complete, the pressure within them begins to fall. This causes the pressure gradient to reverse across the atrioventricular valves, which in turn causes the valves to float upward before closing (Seeley 2000). At this point, the ventricular volumes are at their greatest. The ventricular end-diastolic volume (approximately 120 ml) constitutes the ventricular preload, and is associated with the generation of end-diastolic pressures of 8–12 mmHg in the left ventricles and 3–6 mmHg in the right ventricles (Seeley 2000).

During isovolumetric contraction, all the valves are closed. This phase of the cardiac cycle is initiated by the electrical activity of the conduction system and represents ventricular depolarization. This event (signal) can be picked up on the surface of the body as the QRS complex of the ECG (Seeley 2000). As the ventricles depolarize, a combination of the electrical and chemical events taking place leads to contraction of the myocardium (myocytes) and the development of a tension in the walls of the ventricles with a rapid rise in pressure in the ventricles. Early in this phase, the rate of pressure development is at its maximum. The abrupt rise in pressure causes the atrioventricular valves to close, as the pressure in the ventricles rises above that in the atria. Contraction of the papillary muscles with their attached cordae tendinae prevents the atrioventricular valve flaps from bulging back into the atria and becoming incompetent (allowing blood back into the atria). Closure of the atrioventricular valves can be heard through a stethoscope as the first heart sound (SI). This sound is normally split because the closure of the mitral valve occurs before that of the tricuspid valve (Thibodeau & Patton 2003). During the time between the closure of the atrioventricular valves and the opening of the semilunar valves, the pressure in the ventricles rises rapidly without a change in ventricular volume (no ejection occurs – isovolumetric contraction). Having said that, the contraction of individual myocytes is not necessarily isometric. Individual fibers contract either by shortening (isotonic contraction), by remaining the same length (isometric contraction) or by lengthening (eccentric contraction). As a result, the geometry of the ventricles changes to a more spherical shape with a wider circumference and a shorter length from the base of the atria to the apex of the heart (Seeley 2000, Marieb 2003). The pressure in the atria increases owing to continued venous return combined with potential bulging of the atrioventricular valves back into the atria themselves.

During the rapid ejection phase, the aortic and pulmonary valves are open and the atrioventricular valves remain closed. When the pressure in the ventricles becomes greater

Quiz 1.8

1. Can you describe the mechanical events occurring during atrial systole?

2. Do you know what isovolumetric contraction means?

3. Can you outline the events associated with isovolumetric contraction?

than the pressures within the aorta and pulmonary artery, the aortic and pulmonary valves open and blood is ejected out of the ventricles, and into the systemic and pulmonary circuits (Thibodeau & Patton 2003).

The ejection of blood from the ventricle occurs because the total power of the blood within the ventricle is higher than the total power of blood within the aorta. In other words, there is an energy gradient to propel blood into the aorta and pulmonary artery. During this phase, the pressure in the ventricle is only a few millimeters of mercury higher than that in the aorta. Although blood flow across the valves at this point is very high, the relatively large valve opening, owing to low resistance of the valve, only needs this small pressure gradient to drive flow across the valve. Maximal outpouring velocity is reached early in the ejection phase, and aortic and pulmonary artery (systolic) pressures are at their highest. Heart sounds, in health, are not usually heard during the ejection phase. Pressure in the atria initially falls as the base of the atria is pulled downward, expanding it. Blood continues to flow into the atria from the superior and inferior vena cavae on the right side of the heart, and from the pulmonary veins on the left side of the heart (Seeley 2003).

During the reduced ejection phase, both the aortic and pulmonary valves are open and the atrioventricular valves remain closed. Ventricular repolarization occurs about 150–200 ms after isovolumetric contraction. This event (signal) can be picked up on the surface of the body as the T-wave of the ECG. This causes the dynamic tension in the ventricle to decrease and the ejection rate (ventricular emptying) to fall. Ventricular pressure falls slightly below the pressure in the aorta. Having said that, flow out of the ventricle still takes place. The pressure in the atria rises gradually owing to venous return (Marieb 2003).

During the isovolumetric relaxation phase, all the valves are closed. As the ventricles continue to relax and the pressure in the ventricles falls, a point is reached when the total power of blood within the ventricles is less than the power of blood in the aorta, superior and inferior vena cava (Seeley 2003). At this point, the reversal of pressure causes the aortic and pulmonary valves to close rapidly (the aortic valve closes before the pulmonary valve), causing the second heart sound (S2). When the valves close, a small backflow of blood into the ventricles occurs; this can be seen as a characteristic notch in the aortic and pulmonary artery pressure waveform (we will return to this in Chapter 4). The fall in pressure in the ventricles is not as rapid as the aortic and pulmonary artery pressures. This is because of a potential power or energy that is stored in the walls of the vessels. Because all the valves are closed at this point, the pressure in the ventricle decreases while the volumes do not alter. The pressure in the atria continues to rise owing to the venous return (Marieb 2001).

The volume of ventricular blood that remains in the left ventricle is approximately 50 ml. This is called the end-systolic volume. The difference between the end-diastolic volume and the end-systolic volume is approximately 70 ml. This is the stroke volume. The importance of these terms as monitored values can be found in later chapters of the book.

Quiz 1.9

1. *Can you identify key events that occur during isovolumetric relaxation?*

2. *Do you know what happens to the pressure in the atria and ventricles during the rapid ventricular and reduced ventricular filling phases?*

During the rapid ventricular filling, the atrioventricular valves are open. When the pressure in the ventricles falls below that in the atria, the atrioventricular valves open and ventricular filling begins. Despite this flow of blood into the ventricles, they continue to relax. This causes the pressure in the ventricle to continue to fall by a few additional millimeters of mercury. The opening of the atrioventricular valves brings about a rapid fall in atrial pressures. In individuals with healthy valves, no heart sounds will be heard during filling (Marieb 2001).

During the reduced ventricular filling phase, the ventricles continue to expand as they fill with blood. The pressure in the ventricles rises, as they become less compliant, reducing the pressure gradient across the atrioventricular valves to the extent that the rate of filling falls. During this period, aortic pressure (and pulmonary arterial pressure) continues to fall (Thibodeau & Patton 2003).

Pressure/volume and flow during the cardiac cycle

The pressure in the whole systemic circulation is highest in the aorta and lowest at the point where blood enters the right atrium. As blood is ejected into the aorta by the left ventricle, a characteristic aortic pulse pressure is created (Figure 1.5). The peak of this pressure is the systolic pressure. In contrast, the lowest pressure in the aorta is the diastolic pressure (we will look at the resulting pressure waveform and its interpretation in Chapter 3). The difference between these two pressures (systolic and diastolic) is known as the aortic pulse pressure (Seeley 2000). The average pressure during the aortic pulse cycle is the mean aortic pressure. As the aortic pressure pulse travels down the aorta and into distributing arteries, the systolic, diastolic and mean pressures undergo characteristic changes. As the pulse pressure moves further away from the heart, the systolic pressure rises and the diastolic pressure falls. There is also a small fall in the mean arterial pressure as the pressure pulse travels down into the increasingly divided arteries. Having said that, this fall is relatively insignificant clinically (Thibodeau & Patton 2003). This occurs because of the resistance of the arteries. Obviously, this means that, when arterial pressure is measured, it will always be slightly different from the pressure measurement of the aorta, or the pressure measure in other distributing arteries (Thibodeau & Patton 2003). The relevance of this in relation to monitoring arterial pressures will be discussed in Chapter 4. Venous pressure is the average blood pressure within the venous system. As already discussed, circulatory pressure is at its lowest in the venous system and the pressure gradient from the venules to the right atrium is low (Marieb 2003).

Blood flows throughout the circulatory system because of pressure gradients (Figure 1.6). Pressure is the product of both the volume contained in a chamber and the compliance of the chamber wall. The overall result of blood entering versus blood leaving the chamber determines the volume. Ordinarily blood flow is equal to cardiac output ('flow' and 'cardiac output' are synonymous terms). If the cardiac output is increased, it follows that the flow of blood through the capillary bed will also increase.

During the cardiac cycle just prior to contraction, the pressure in the ventricle is less than the venous return. This

Quiz 1.10

1. *Can you define arterial blood pressure?*
2. *Can you define venous return?*

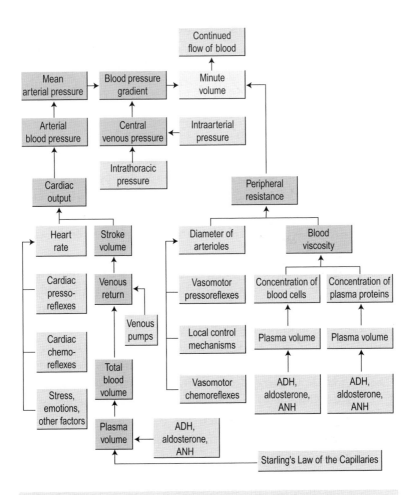

Fig 1.6 Factors that influence the flow of blood. This chart shows some of the main influences on blood flow. Some of these factors affect blood flow in more than one way, as demonstrated in the chart. ADH, antidiuretic hormone; ANP, antinatriuretic peptide. (Reproduced with permission from Thibodeau & Patton 2003).

causes blood to flow into the ventricle because of the pressure gradient (Seeley 2000). The walls of the ventricle are very compliant (low resistance) so the volume entering does not cause a great increase in pressure. Having said that, as the wall is stretched further, it becomes less compliant

Quiz 1.11

1. *Do you know what determines blood flow?*

2. *Can you describe the flow, pressure and volume changes in the heart during the cardiac cycle?*

(more resistant), so there is a greater rise in pressure if the volume increases (Seeley 2000). As the myocardium contracts, the pressure in the ventricles rises, but the volume stays the same. This is because increased elastance of the fibers increases its ability to stretch (up to a point).

During the ejection phase of the cardiac cycle, the volume in the ventricles is decreasing (blood is being ejected out across the aortic valve into the systemic circulation). At the same time, the pressure is rising slightly, and then falls. As pressure and volume are changing, the elastance of the myocardium continues to increase (from the beginning of systole to the end of systole). It is the changes occurring at cellular level that alter the mechanical properties of the muscle, making it stiffer (less compliant). At the end of systole, the pressure falls abruptly while the volume remains the same. This is because the elastance is decreasing. Pressure and resistance in the cardiovascular system directly affects the afterload of the heart (the resistance that the ventricle has to eject against). Having said that, if there was no resistance to blood flow, the heart would not have to generate pressure to force blood around the pulmonary and systemic circuits (Tortora & Grabowski 2003).

The electrocardiogram

The specialized structures of the heart's conduction system generate tiny electrical currents that spread throughout surrounding tissues to the surface of the body (Figure 1.5). These electrical signals can then be picked up from the body surface and transformed into visible tracings by an electro-cardiogram, otherwise known as the ECG (Thaler 2003, Thibodeau & Patton 2003). This graphical record of the electrical events occurring in the heart has three very characteristic deflections or waves, called the P-wave, QRS complex and the T-wave (Figure 1.5). These represent the electrical activity that regulates the contraction or relaxation of the atria and ventricles. By comparing the information obtained from electrodes placed at different locations, the electrical activity of the heart in relation to nodal, con-ducting and contractile components can be evaluated (Thibodeau & Patton 2003). We will return to this in more detail in further sections of the book.

Quiz 1.12

1. *What is an ECG?*

2. *Can you identify the characteristic deflections that represent the electrical events occurring in the heart?*

TERMINOLOGY BOX 1.2

Depolarization – The reduction of voltage across a plasma membrane towards less negative (more positive) voltage on the interior surface of the plasma membrane

Repolarization – The restoration of the voltages that existed across the plasma membrane before depolarization took place

Action potential – An electrical signal that propagates along the membrane of a neuron or muscle fiber that involves depolarization followed by repolarization

REFERENCES

Brooker C G 1993 Human structure and function nursing applications in clinical practice. Mosby, St Louis, MO

Darovic G O 2002 Hemodynamic monitoring: invasive and noninvasive clinical applications, 3rd edn. Saunders

Marieb E N 2001 Human anatomy and physiology, 5th edn. Benjamin Cummings, San Francisco

Marieb E N 2003 Essentials of human anatomy and physiology, 7th edn. Addison Wesley Longman, Harlow

Rutishauser S 1997 Physiology and anatomy: a basis for nursing and health care, 2nd edn. Churchill Livingstone, Edinburgh

Saladin K 1997 Anatomy and physiology: the unity of form and function. WCB McGraw-Hill, California

Seeley R R 2000 Anatomy and physiology, 5th edn. WCB McGraw-Hill, California

Solomon E, Davies P 1996 Anatomy and physiology, 4th edn. Mosby, St Louis, MO

Thaler M S 2003 The only EKG book you'll ever need. Lippincott Williams and Wilkins, Philadelphia

Thibodeau G A, Patton K T 2003 Anatomy and physiology, 5th edn. Mosby, St Louis, MO

Tortora G J, Grabowski S R 2003 Principles of anatomy and physiology, 10th edn, John Wiley, New York

SUGGESTED READING

Berne R M, Levy, M N 2001 Cardiovascular physiology, 8th edn. Mosby, St Louis, MO

Criner G J, Alonzo E D !999 Pulmonary pathophysiology. Blackwell Science, Oxford

Kusumoto F M 1999 Cardiovascular pathophysiology. Blackwell Science, Oxford

Marieb E N 2001 Fundamentals of anatomy and physiology, 5th edn. Prentice Hall, New Jersey

Martini F H 2001 Fundamentals of anatomy and physiology, 5th edn. Prentice Hall, New Jersey

2 Cardiodynamics

Main objectives

- State what cardiac output is, how it is controlled and regulated, and describe the factors that affect it.
- Explain the meaning of the terms preload, afterload and contractility.
- Explain the relationship between oxygen supply, demand and extraction, and their relationship to tissue perfusion
- Explain the mechanisms involved in the regulation of blood flow, and how blood pressure is controlled and regulated.

Introduction

For survival, the body needs to be able to extract oxygen not only from the atmosphere but also to be able to transport it to its cells in order to utilize it for metabolic processes. Most cells are able to produce energy without the need to use oxygen (anaerobic metabolism) but only for a short time, and the process is not particularly efficient (Tortora & Grabowski 2003). Organs, such as the brain, are made up of cells that are only able to produce the energy they require to survive and only in the presence of a constant supply of oxygen (aerobic metabolism). The ability to withstand anoxia (lack of oxygen) differs from tissue to tissue (Seeley 2000). However, both the brain and the heart are by far the most sensitive. A lack of oxygen initially affects the function of organs. However, in time, damage that is irreversible is done; in the case of the brain, this occurs in minutes (Marieb 2003).

Optimization or goal-directed therapy, as it is otherwise known (we return to this subject in detail in Chapter 7), aims to utilize what we know about the normal function of the cardiovascular system (cardiodynamics) and manipulate its component parts in order to improve the chances of survival for critically ill patients.

Cardiac output

The amount of blood ejected from a ventricle during a single heartbeat is the stroke volume. The amount of blood pumped by a ventricle each minute is the cardiac output (Darovic 2002). The cardiac output (CO) is the product of stroke volume (SV) and heart rate (HR): The cardiac index (CI) is the cardiac output per square meter of body surface area and is a normalizing technique used to compare cardiac outputs of different-sized individuals. Cardiac index tends to be used more frequently clinically. The cardiac output provides a good indication of ventricular efficiency over time (Darovic 2002). We will consider each of these components in more detail.

Stroke volume

The stroke volume is the most important factor when looking at a single heart cycle because it tells us how much blood is being ejected from the ventricle with every heartbeat. Factors that affect stroke volume include the end-diastolic volume, the end-systolic volume, contractility and autonomic activity (Thibodeau & Patten 2003). The largest stroke volume is achieved when the end-diastolic volume is as high as it can be and the end-systolic volume is as small as it can be. End-diastolic volume is affected by two factors: filling time, which depends entirely on heart rate – the higher the rate, the shorter the filling time; and the venous return, which is affected by alterations in cardiac output, blood volume, patterns of peripheral circulation, skeletal muscle activity, etc.

Quiz 2.1

1. What is cardiac output and cardiac index?

2. What factors can affect stroke volume?

3. Can you say which two factors affect end-diastolic volume?

TERMINOLOGY BOX 2.1

End-diastolic volume (EDV) – The amount of blood in each ventricle at the end of ventricular diastole (or start of systole)

End-systolic volume (ESV) – The amount of blood remaining in each ventricle at the end of ventricular systole (the start of ventricular diastole)

Stroke volume (SV) – The amount of blood pumped out of each ventricle during a single beat, which can be expressed as:

EDV − ESV = SV

Ejection fraction – The percentage of the EDV represented by the stroke volume

Preload

Preload is the amount of tension on the cardiac muscle before it begins to contract (systole). The more they are stretched (to a certain point, and we will come back to this), the stronger is the contraction that occurs during systole, and, therefore, the greater is the stroke volume. This relationship between ventricular end-diastolic volume and stroke volume is known as the Frank–Starling law of the heart, which states that the energy of contraction of the muscle is related/proportional to the initial length of the muscle fiber (Tortora & Grabowski 2003). The more blood there is in the chamber just prior to systole (at the end of diastole), the greater the stretch. The end-diastolic volume is the amount of blood found in the ventricle at the end of diastole. This is the greatest amount of blood found in the ventricle during the cardiac cycle. Preload is mainly dependent on the return of blood from the body (venous return). Venous return is influenced by changes in position, intrathoracic pressure, blood volume and the balance of constriction and dilation (tone) in the venous system (Marieb 2003).

Contractility

Contractility describes the ability of the myocardium to contract in the absence of any changes in preload or after-

---

Quiz 2.2

1. Do you know what preload is?

2. Can you outline Frank–Starling's law?

3. What is the end-diastolic volume?

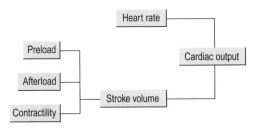

Fig 2.1 Determinants of stroke volume and cardiac output. (Reproduced with permission from Darovic 2002.)

load. In other words, it is the intrinsic (physical) strength of the ventricle, independent of loading conditions (Seeley 2000). The most important influence on contractility is the sympathetic nervous system. Beta-adrenergic receptors in the myocardium are stimulated by noradrenaline (see Chapter 1) released from nerve endings, and contractility is increased. If everything was kept in a constant state and contractility was increased (let's say by epinephrine release, for example), the ventricle would empty more of its contents during ejection; therefore, stroke volume would increase (Darovic 2002). If the preload and afterload are unchanged, raising contractility increases stroke volume. Lowering contractility decreases stroke volume (Figure 2.1; Thibodeau & Patten 2003).

Afterload

Before the ventricle can start to move blood through the aortic valve, the pressure in the ventricle must equal that in the aorta. The forces that oppose ejection of blood out of the ventricles or, in other words, the 'resistance' to ventricular ejection, are caused by the resistance to flow in the systemic

> ## Quiz 2.3
>
> 1. Can you define myocardial contractility?
> 2. Do you know which neurotransmitter affects contractility?
> 3. Can you briefly explain what afterload is?

circulation. This is the systemic vascular resistance. The resistance is determined by the diameter of the arterioles and pre-capillary sphincters (Thibodeau & Patten 2003). The narrower and more constricted these vessels, the higher the resistance. The level of systemic vascular resistance is controlled by the sympathetic nervous system, which in turn controls the tone of the muscle in the walls of the arterioles and, therefore, the diameter (Thibodeau & Patten 2003). Under normal conditions, the heart does not eject all of its contents. It normally ejects approximately two-thirds of the blood that is in the ventricle at end-diastole (i.e. the normal ejection fraction is approximately 67%).

If afterload were increased, less of the blood in the ventricle would be ejected, reducing the cardiac output (Darovic 2002). If afterload were decreased, more of the blood in the ventricle would be ejected, increasing cardiac output. Therefore, in a steady state, raising afterload decreases stroke volume and lowering afterload increases it.

Heart rate

The heart rate is determined by the rate of spontaneous depolarization at the sinoatrial node, modified by the autonomic nervous system (cardioaccelerator/cardioinhibitory center in the medulla). Factors that affect the heart rate include autonomic innervation (the sympathetic and parasympathetic nerve supply to the myocardium), cardiac reflexes, autonomic tone, effects on the sinoatrial node, the atrial reflex, hormones (such as epinephrine and norepinephrine), and the venous return (Mark 1998).

The vagus nerve acts on receptors to slow the heart rate, whereas the cardiac sympathetic fibers stimulate beta-adrenergic receptors to increase it (by changing cell membrane permeability in the conducting system). These cardiac centers receive input from higher centers and from baroreceptors (sensing pressure) and chemoreceptors (detecting changes in chemical concentrations). On the basis of information received, cardiac performance is adjusted, responding to changes in blood pressure and arterial concentrations of dissolved oxygen (O_2) and carbon dioxide (CO_2). Acetylcholine (parasympathetic nervous system hormone) acts by opening chemically gated K^+ channels slowing the rate of spontaneous depolarization (reduction of voltage across the membrane) and extending the period of repolarization (restoration of voltage across the membrane). Norepinephrine works by binding to beta-1 receptors leading to the opening of Ca^{2+} channels increasing the rate of depolarization and shortening repolarization. The atrial reflex accelerates the heart rate when the arterial walls are stretched (Marieb 2003).

Quiz 2.4

1. *Do you know what determines heart rate?*

2. *Can you identify the factors that can affect heart rate?*

3. *Can you say which neurotransmitters are involved in the regulation of afterload?*

4. *Can you say which receptors are involved and what they do?*

A decrease in cardiac output can occur for many reasons. Decreases in heart rate or the loss of contractility (e.g. ventricular failure) cause blood to back up into the venous circulation, causing an increase in venous volume. This is as a result of less blood being pumped into the arterial circulation. In turn, this causes an increase in thoracic blood volume, resulting in an increased central venous pressure. In renal failure, or when the renin–angiotensin–aldosterone system is activated, an increase in the total volume of blood occurs and results in an increase in venous pressure. Sympathetic activation of veins and circulating vasoconstrictor substances (e.g. catecholamines and angiotensin II) brings about venous constriction, decreasing the compliance of the venous system and increasing venous pressure. When the patient changes position (e.g. from supine to standing), a shift in blood volume into the thoracic venous compartment occurs and increases central venous pressure. Arterial vasodilator drugs cause an increase in blood flow from the arterial into the venous systems. This results in an increase in the venous volume and, therefore, the pressure. This also occurs when sympathetic tone is reduced. This is true when the heart is functioning normally. However, in ventricular failure, arterial dilation brings about a decrease in venous pressure. This is because arterial dilation reduces the afterload on the ventricle, increasing stroke volume. In ventricular failure, stroke volume is more strongly affected by afterload. Central venous pressure is also increased during a forced expiration (e.g. during a Valsalva maneuver). The pressure in the venous system rises because external compression of the thoracic vena cava occurs as intrathoracic pressure rises. Veins are compressed during muscle contraction (more in the limbs and abdomen) causing a decrease in compliance and forcing blood into the thorax (Rutishauser 1997, Mark 1998, Marieb 2003).

The control of cardiac output

Cardiac output can be adjusted by changes in either heart rate or stroke volume. However, having said that, changes in cardiac output generally reflect changes in both heart rate and stroke volume (Darovic 2002). The heart rate can be adjusted by the activities of the autonomic nervous system or by circulating hormones (as already discussed). Venous return has an indirect effect on the heart rate by atrial reflexes (accelerates the heart rate when the arterial walls are stretched). It also has a direct effect on the cells of the nodes. When venous return increases, the atria receive more blood and the walls are stretched. This stretching of the cells of the sinoatrial node leads to more rapid depolarization and an increase in heart rate (Seeley 2000). The stroke volume can be adjusted by changing the end-diastolic volume (how full the ventricles are when they start to contract), the end-systolic volume (how much blood remains in the ventricle after it contracts), or both. In this way, the cardiovascular system responds to the changing needs of the tissues for oxygen (Marieb 2003).

Oxygen delivery

The oxygen delivery (DO_2) is the amount of oxygen delivered to the tissues bound to hemoglobin. The ability of the

Quiz 2.5

1. *In order to control cardiac output do you know how is it adjusted?*

2. *Do you know how the heart rate adjusted?*

3. *Can you say how the stroke volume adjusted?*

body to produce energy (mainly ATP – energy) using aerobic (oxygen utilization) cellular metabolism is a fundamental physiological process. Normal cellular function and homeostatic processes depend on this more efficient method of producing energy for survival. For example, it is worth noting that aerobic metabolism is able to produce 38 molecules of ATP for every single molecule of glucose, whereas anaerobic metabolism is only able to produce two. In order for aerobic metabolism to occur, oxygen must be delivered to the tissues and cells, where it can be processed by the mitochondria (Seeley 2000, Thibodeau & Patten 2003).

The oxygen delivery is a derived value. In order to calculate it, the equation requires information about the oxygen content of arterial blood and the flow of blood leaving the left side of the heart (cardiac output). Therefore, the oxygen delivery is equal to the cardiac output multiplied by the oxygen content of arterial blood.

Therefore, it can be seen that oxygen delivery is not only dependent on the efficient exchange of gases in the lungs (to take in oxygen), adequate levels of hemoglobin (for oxygen to bind to) and the ability of oxygen to bind with it (quality of the hemoglobin itself), but also on an adequate cardiac output (flow of blood; Leach & Treacher 2002, Hameed et al 2003, Walsh 2003).

The transfer of oxygen from the atmosphere to the mitochondria is dependent upon two processes: convection and diffusion. Air transfers from the atmosphere to the alveoli by convection and then diffuses across the alveolar membrane in the alveoli into the red cells. Once combined with oxygen, convective movement carries oxyhemoglobin to the tissues, where oxygen diffuses out of the red cell into the mitochondria (Marieb 2003). Ordinarily, the supply of oxygen (DO_2) to the tissues is higher than that of consumption (VO_2). Having said that, during critical illness (or exercise and at high altitudes), the oxygen supply may not be adequate to meet demand and tissue hypoxia will occur. A great deal of attention is being focused on the adequate supply of oxygen to the tissues because of its proven influence on mortality, morbidity and length of hospital stay, and the maintenance of an adequate level of oxygen delivery is now accepted as essential in the care of the critically ill patient. However, there is little agreement on what the level of DO_2 should be. In addition, in certain situations, despite apparently sufficient oxygen delivery, factors such as extracellular and intracellular edema and dysfunction at mitochondrial level will inevitably impair oxygen utilization. Delivery of adequate amounts of oxygen does not guarantee the ability of the tissues to utilize it (Darovic 2002).

Oxygen consumption

Oxygen consumption (VO_2) is the amount of oxygen extracted from hemoglobin and utilized by all body cells, in order to carry out normal metabolic processes. Some conditions actually limit tissue oxygen consumption to a level that is below that demanded by the tissues. Conditions that produce abnormal capillary blood flow, such as acute respiratory distress syndrome (ARDS), sepsis and septic shock, limit the oxygen consumption to a level that is far less than that being demanded. This creates an oxygen debt (Figure 2.2). If this oxygen debt continues over time, organ dysfunction is inevitable and survival unlikely (Darovic 2002). A patient who has a very low oxygen delivery and a high metabolic rate (e.g. because of increased work of breathing or agitation) would not be able to consume sufficient oxygen to meet the demands of the

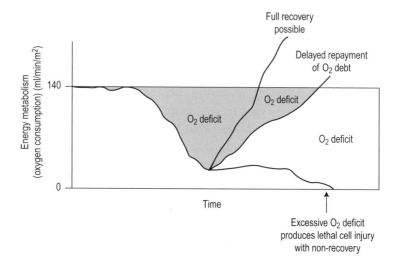

Fig 2.2 Oxygen debt occurs when there is not enough oxygen delivery to meet the requirements for energy metabolism. If the debt is significant but repaid, full recovery is possible. If delayed repayment results, then there can be organ dysfunction and, much worse, death can result.

tissues. Tissues and cells that do not receive blood flow (because of maldistribution) are unable to consume enough oxygen to meet demand.

Myocardial oxygen consumption is primarily determined by contracting cells. Anything that increases the rate of contraction (tension development) or the amount of contractions (rate), results in an increase in the oxygen demand of the myocardium. For example, if the heart rate doubles, it will follow that the myocardial oxygen consumption will also double. This is because the ventricular cells (myocytes) are generating twice the number of cycles per minute. In addition, increasing contractility also increases myocardial oxygen consumption (Seeley 2000). This is because the rate of contraction development is increased as well as the degree of contractility. Both of these increase energy utilization and, therefore, oxygen consumption. Contractility can be increased by increasing the afterload, which then in turn increases myocardial oxygen consumption. In addition, increasing preload also increases myocardial oxygen consumption. Having said that, the increase is not as great as you might expect. This is because myocardial wall tension is proportional to the pressure in the ventricle and its radius. This is known as the 'La Place' relationship (Darovic 2002).

The tension of the heart wall is the amount of tension created by the myocytes (myocardial cells) that results in a degree of pressure within the ventricle at a given radius. So, for example, when the ventricle has to generate a greater pressure in order to overcome an increased afterload, the wall tension rises. Wall tension and, therefore, myocardial oxygen consumption is far less sensitive to changes in ventricular volume than pressure (Figure 2.3).

Oxygen demand

Oxygen demand is closely related to the oxygen consumption of an organ. Although they are not the same thing (see later section on 'Oxygen extraction'), they are often used interchangeably. Oxygen demand is related to need. On the other hand, oxygen consumption is the actual amount of oxygen consumed per minute of time (Darovic 2002). Under certain conditions, demand is greater than consumption, simply because the delivery of oxygen to the heart is limited for some reason.

The heart does have a high demand for oxygen and, therefore, consumes high amounts. The oxygen consumption of

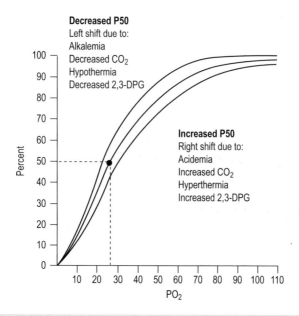

Fig 2.3 Oxyhemoglobin dissociation curve showing how the affinity of hemoglobin changes with temperature, CO_2 and the pH of the blood. (Reproduced with permission from Darovic 2002.)

the myocardium (MVO_2), for example, is necessary in order to generate energy (ATP). This energy is then utilized by cell membrane transport mechanisms, such as the Na^+/K^+ pump, and by the contracting and relaxing of the cells (Marieb 2003). When the heart is at rest, the myocardium consumes approximately 8 ml/min per g, whereas, when the heart is working hard (e.g. during exercise), it consumes approximately 70 ml of oxygen/min per g. When this is compared to other organs in the body (i.e. the kidneys, brain and contracting skeletal muscles), its oxygen consumption is considerably higher.

During times when demand for oxygen is increased, the heart has to extract more oxygen from the blood supplying the myocardium in order to support oxygen consumption adequately (Seeley 2000). Meanwhile, the nervous system responds by trying to increase the oxygen delivery. The relationship between myocardial oxygen consumption, coronary blood flow and the amount of oxygen extracted from the blood (arteriovenous oxygen difference) is unique and is an application of the Fick principle, which we will return to in a later chapter (Thibodeau & Patten 2003).

Oxygen extraction (SvO_2)

The oxygen saturation of venous blood is a reflection of oxygen return to the right side of the heart. Ordinarily, this would be 75%, with the normal range being 60% to 80%. When the body is at rest, approximately 600 ml/min per m^2 is delivered to the tissues, and they consume 150 ml/min per m^2, which represents the basal metabolic rate. Blood then flows back to the heart at the approximate rate of 450 ml/min per m^2 (varies with age). Therefore, the oxygen delivery (DO_2) is four times the oxygen consumption (VO_2) – 600 ml:150 ml; therefore, the balance between supply and demand is 4:1, with an extraction of oxygen of 25% (Kusumoto 1999, White 2003).

If the body is demanding more oxygen for any reason (and the critically ill patient will be), the central nervous system responds by increasing the oxygen delivery in order to maintain the 4:1 balance between supply and demand. However, in patients unable to respond by increasing oxygen delivery, the extraction of oxygen then increases, and can be considerable. For example, if the oxygen delivery falls to 255 ml/min per m^2, the venous oxygen saturation would fall to 39% (in patients who ordinarily have a normal resting metabolic rate). A prolonged imbalance between supply and demand and low venous oxygen saturations is an ominous sign, and is associated with a poor outcome (Lake et al 2001, White 2003).

If the venous oxygen saturation is less than 75%, the oxygen consumption is below normal. Having said that, at this point, there could still be shunting of peripheral blood flow, which is undetectable. At 50%, the balance between supply and demand has fallen to 2:1, and a venous oxygen saturation less than 35% indicates that anaerobic metabolism is already occurring in the tissues and symptoms of organ dysfunction will be apparent (Criner & Alonzo 1999, Lakadis et al 2001).

There are many causes of increases and decreases in tissue oxygen demand. It should be noted that many of these are as a result of nursing interventions and clinical routines. For example, having visitors can increase oxygen demand by 22% and getting a patient out of bed into a chair can increase it by 40–50%. A bed bath can increase oxygen demand by 23%, while turning the patient can increase it by 31% (White 2003). Treating a low oxygen delivery is important but oxygen demand should be reduced where possible. Unfortunately, oxygen demand cannot be measured. Having said that, it can be estimated from the patients resting metabolic rate, the work of breathing and the oxygen consumption (Kusumoto 1999, Tisherman 2000).

REFERENCES

Criner G J, Alonzo E D 1999 Pulmonary pathophysiology. Blackwell Science, Oxford

Darovic G O 2002 Hemodynamic monitoring: invasive and non-invasive clinical applications, 3rd edn. Saunders, Philadelphia

Hameed S M, Aird W E, Cohn S M 2003 Oxygen delivery. Critical Care Medicine 31(Suppl 12): S658–S667

Kusumoto F M 1999 Cardiovascular pathophysiology. Blackwell Science, Oxford

Ladakis C, Myrianthefs P, Karabinis A et al 2001 Central venous and mixed venous oxygen saturation in critically ill patients. Respiration 68: 279–285

Lake C L, Hines R L, Blitt C D 2001 Clinical monitoring: practical applications for anaesthesia and critical care. Saunders, Philadelphia

Leach R M, Treacher D F 2002 The pulmonary physician in critical care: oxygen delivery and consumption in the critically ill. Thorax 57: 170–177

Marieb E N 2003 Essentials of human anatomy and physiology, 7th edn. Addison Wesley Longman, Harlow

Mark J B 1998 Atlas of cardiovascular monitoring. Churchill Livingstone, Edinburgh

Rutishauser S 1997 Physiology and anatomy: a basis for nursing and health care, 2nd edn. Churchill Livingstone, Edinburgh

Seeley R R 2000 Anatomy and physiology, 5th edn. WCB McGraw-Hill, California

Thibodeau G A, Patten K T 2003 Anatomy and physiology, 5th edn. Mosby, St Louis, MO

Tisherman S A 2000 Postinjury oxygen consumption. New methods, no new answers. Critical Care Medicine 28: 577–578

Tortora G J, Grabowski S R 2003 Principles of anatomy and physiology, 10th edn. John Wiley, New York

Walsh T A 2003 Recent advances in gas exchange measurement in intensive care unit patients. British Journal of Anaesthesia 91: 120–131

White K 2003 Fast facts for adult critical care. Kathy White Learning Systems, Alabama

SUGGESTED READING

Berne R M, Levy M N 2001 Cardiovascular physiology, 8th edn. Mosby, St Louis, MO

Criner G J, Alonzo E D 1999 Pulmonary pathophysiology. Blackwell Science, Oxford

Edwards J D 1990 Practical application of oxygen transport principles. Critical Care Medicine 18:S45-S48

Edwards J D 1991 Oxygen transport in cardiogenic and septic shock. Critical Care Medicine 19: 658–663

Hayes M A, Timmins A C, Yau E H, Palazoo M, Hindo C J, Watson D 1994 Evaluation of systemic oxygen delivery in the treatment of the critically ill. New England Journal of Medicine 330: 1717–1722

Kusumoto F M 1999 Cardiovascular pathophysiology. Blackwell Science, Oxford

Marieb E N 2001 Fundamentals of anatomy and physiology, 5th edn. Prentice Hall, New Jersey

Martini F H 2001 Fundamentals of anatomy and physiology, 5th edn. Prentice Hall, New Jersey

Pinsky M R 1994 Beyond global oxygen supply-demand relations: in search of measures of dysoxia. Intensive Care Medicine 20: 1–3

Pinsky M R 2002 Functional hemodynamic monitoring. Intensive Care Medicine 28: 386–388

Reinhart K, Kuhn H J, Hartog C, Bredle D L 2004 Continuous central venous and pulmonary artery saturation monitoring in the critically ill. Intensive Care Medicine (epub ahead of print)

Van de Louw A, Cracco C, Cerf C et al 2001 Accuracy of pulse oximetry in the intensive care unit. Intensive Care Medicine 27: 1606–1613

3 Back to basics: hemodynamic monitoring

Types of monitoring system

For invasive pressure monitoring, most intensive care units use disposable sets (single, double or, in some cases, multiple), comprising a pressure transducer and consistently compliant extension tubing (this is an important point), which is then connected to an intravascular catheter (Darovic 2002). The whole system is then filled with fluid (usually saline but not always, and each intensive care unit will vary in its policies). A cable then links up to an electronic amplifier monitor from this fluid-filled set. The system works by pulsatile pressure at the tip of the catheter (from inside the patient), being transmitted through the connecting tubing (which is filled with fluid) to the diaphragm of the transducer. The movement of the transducer diaphragm (which is induced by pressure) is then converted into electrical signals that are of a low voltage (Mark 1998). These pressure signals are then amplified and converted by the amplifier and monitor into a continuous waveform and digital value on an oscilloscope. An oscilloscope allows the amplified pulse pressure wave to be viewed continuously as the events are occurring (Mark 1998).

Getting the most accurate information from your fluid-filled system

For several reasons, it is important to be familiar with the physical characteristics of fluid-filled pressure monitoring systems. Firstly, it is routine in intensive care units to use fluid-filled catheter/transducer systems for hemodynamic monitoring. Secondly, these monitoring systems have unique characteristics, and distorted waveforms and inaccurate pressure measurements can be controlled with an awareness of the factors that contribute to them. The pressure displayed by bedside monitors is taken from compartments of the cardiovascular system to allow for cardiovascular function assessment (Mark 1998, Darovic 2002).

The underlying principle of current methods of invasive monitoring is that, at any point in an unobstructed system, a change in pressure results in a pressure change that is similar at other points in the system. A fluid medium is difficult to compress. This fact allows the accurate transmission of pressure from the catheter tip (which is located in the patient's body) to an amplifier/monitor that is zeroed and calibrated (we will come to this later; Mark 1998, Darovic 2002).

Pressure transducers

Pressure transducers are electromechanical devices that detect pressure and convert that pressure into an electrical signal. Of the different types of pressure transducers that are available for use in intensive care units, the pretested, calibrated and sterilized disposable transducers are used most commonly. This is because they are smaller in size, less expensive, more robust and, importantly, more accurate (Darovic 2002, Tang et al 2002).

They all have a diaphragm, which is pressure sensitive, enclosed by a dome that is then filled with fluid. Pressure pulsations detected from the patient are transmitted by the fluid and make contact with the diaphragm. The movement of the diaphragm is then converted into an electrical signal, which is then processed and displayed on the monitor/amplifier (Mark 1998, Thevenot et al 2001, Darovic 2002, Bhatia & Mackenzie 2004).

As other authors have pointed out previously (Mark 1998), 'ducer' (from 'transducer') means to mislead, calculate or to draw along, and is probably worth remembering when you are not sure whether to believe the readings you are getting! Measurements should always be taken in the context of the whole picture and not just as isolated readings (Barbireri & Kaplan 1983).

It is important that the amplifier is able to take a signal (e.g. 1 mV) and reproduce it, so that it is displayed consistently ten times that of the original signal. This ensures that a

Quiz 3.1

1. *What are the important parameters in a catheter–transducer system?*

2. *Do you know what an underdamped trace is caused by?*

3. *Do you know what an overdamped trace is caused by?*

pressure reading of, say 100 mmHg, would appear as a waveform that would be exactly twice that of a pressure reading of 50 mmHg. This is an important requirement because it allows judgements to be made about changes in both waveform height and the digital readings based on accurate pressures. Having said that, the system also needs to be correctly leveled and zeroed (Rolfe 1990, Baker & Gough 1996, Mark 1998, Darovic 2002).

In addition, the amplifier must be able to respond to changes in pressure quickly and with accuracy, if it is to be of any value. Most current monitoring systems are able to respond to changes in pressure within milliseconds. Obviously, the shorter the time it takes from the actual event and the data being displayed on the monitor the better, so that accurate timing of events that occur can be made.

In order for accurate pressure measurements to be displayed, the whole fluid-filled transducer system has to be unobstructed, zero referenced and leveled (we return to this later in the chapter). The fluid-filled components of the system are connected to a flush device that is ordinarily mounted on the transducer itself. An intravenous fluid bag from which the set has been primed (which usually comes as part of a ready-packaged set) is then put under pressure using an inflatable pressure bag. This ensures that the system remains patent. For an adult, a pressure of 300 mmHg is sufficient to maintain the patency of the system by delivering a counter pressure against the pulsatile pressure coming from the venous or arterial line in the patient. This amounts to the continuous infusion of approximately 3 ml of fluid per hour.

The use of prepacked transducer sets for invasive pressure monitoring, which usually contains all the necessary components required, not only reduces the risk of contamination because the sets are fully assembled (and ready to be primed and connected), but also increases the reliability of the pressure measurements generated. This is because the transducer and all the other components of the system (i.e. compliance and length of the tubing) have been factory set (Mark 1998, Darovic 2002).

It is sometimes common practice for an additional amount of tubing to be added into the arterial line circuit to give a longer length of tubing and, therefore, provide easier access to the stopcocks. This is particularly true in surgical patients during the operative procedure. The problem with this is that the transducer set has been calibrated to take into account not only the length of the tubing but also its compliance. These have initially been taken into account when calibrating the dynamic response of the whole set. Adding additional tubing that does not comply with the diameter or compliance of the original tubing compromises the accuracy of the information subsequently gained. Transducer sets with longer tubing are available and these are a much better option.

The supine position is thought of as the standard position for the patient to be in for pressure measurement. This is because the hemodynamic values that we consider to be normal were obtained from healthy subjects who happened to be in the supine position (Mark 1998). It should be noted that raising or lowering the patient's head and chest does affect the accuracy of pressure measurement. This is because of the effects of gravity on blood flow and, therefore, intravascular pressure. Having said that, if the thorax is elevated to 30–40°, there would not be a clinically significant change (Mark 1998).

In some cases, patients are unable to tolerate the supine or 40° raised position for very long (i.e. breathless patients, and those with chronic obstructive pulmonary disease or heart failure). However, it is important to take into account that measurements may be less than those recorded from the supine position. As with all measurements, trends over time are more important than single or absolute values. In order for any hemodynamic measurements to have any meaning, any change in the way the measurements are made or the position the patient is in at the time should be noted, so that everyone is aware. For example, 'in this patient, supine position is being used for all measurement', and then clearly document any deviation from this, if there is a change in any measured variable. This can then be taken into account (Mark 1998).

Water manometers

Water manometer monitoring systems utilize an existing central venous catheter that is attached to fluid-filled connecting tubing and then to a water manometer (Lake et al 2001). It is a simple way of measuring the central venous pressure that is frequently used in hospital ward areas, where the use of transducers is uncommon.

The system comprises of an upside-down, T-shaped, fluid-filled catheter that is attached to the central line at one end and a bag of fluid (usually saline) at the other. The T-component of the catheter is attached vertically to a water manometer mounting plate. This has increments in centimetres of water (cmH_2O) written on it. This part of the catheter has a filter at its tip. When the connection between the patient and the catheter is unobstructed, the pressure in the venous system causes the column of water to rise. When it comes to rest at some point on the manometer, the cmH_2O reading is taken as being the central venous pressure (pressure required to raise the column of water to that level).

Water manometer monitoring systems do have drawbacks. For example, the measurements are only intermittent and they have to be obtained manually. Often measurements cannot be made owing to accidental overflow of fluid from the manometer tip during the priming process. This is usually because the tap in the system has been turned in the wrong direction, directly filling the T-section from the bag of fluid, rather that flushing fluid into the central venous catheter. This can cause a backflow of potentially contaminated fluid into the system (Mark 1998).

As the measuring units used by water manometers are cmH_2O, which is different from the units used to obtain other monitored parameters (usually mmHg), it can be difficult to make comparisons (Darovic 2002).

Is my pressure monitoring reliable?

Fluid-filled monitoring systems have certain physical properties that can affect the faithful reproduction of both the pressure measurement and the waveform shape. These properties need to be taken into account when interpreting generated data. Dynamic response testing (Gardner 1981, Gardner & Hollingsworth 1986, Tang et al 2002) allows us to test the system's ability to reproduce pressure pulse sensed (Figure 3.1) from the patient to the monitor/amplifier accurately. Dynamic response is related to the relationship between the natural frequencies of the system itself, the pressure signals being detected and the amount of damping that is present. The simplest way of doing this is with a square wave test (fast flush test; Box 3.1; Mark 1998, Darovic 2002, D'Orazio 2003).

If carried out with low-compliant, continuous-flush devices (as prepacked transducer sets are), it will enable the

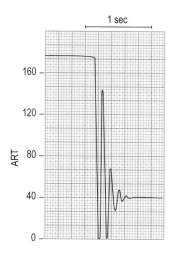

Fig 3.1 Dynamic response testing using the fast flush fluid system. (Reproduced with permission from Mark 1998.)

Box 3.1 Measuring natural frequency and damping coefficient

The ability to perform a fast flush test provides a rapid method to distinguish true arterial hypotension from artifactual hypotension caused by a large air bubble or blood clot in the catheter or tubing

Method

1. Open the fast-flush valve several times (preferably during diastolic runoff so that the flush signal is not distorted by the systolic arterial pressure upstroke or dicrotic notch)
2. Examine the resulting artifact

---

determination of the natural frequency, the damping characteristics, and whether they are able to produce accurate waveforms and digital values faithfully. It should be remembered that a simple system is much more likely to give accurate information than a system that is complex (i.e. additional tubing, three way taps, etc.). In order to have the highest natural frequency and the minimum amount of damping, short stiff catheters are recommended (Gardner

& Hollingsworth 1986). In addition, the distance between the catheter and the transducer should be as short as possible with a large internal diameter both for the tubing and the catheter (whether it is an arterial, central or pulmonary artery catheter). When setting up the system, care should be taken to remove all air bubbles from the tubing and stopcocks, as this can also affect accuracy (Shinozaki et al 1980).

Leveling

Having zeroed the transducer to the atmosphere, it is then just as important to have the transducer at the correct level. Leveling is required because, from the tip of the catheter to the pressure measurement device, it is filled with fluid. A hydrostatic pressure from the mid-chest to the measuring device, against the transducer diaphragm (or water manometer), can either add or subtract from the real pressure measured. In the majority of cases, the tip of a catheter put in for central pressure monitoring (including a pulmonary artery catheter) is approximately at mid-chest level or the phlebostatic axis (one-half of the anterior-posterior diameter) of the patient just below the angle of the sternum (White 2003). This position was chosen because examination using a fluoroscope shows that, with the patient in the supine position, the left ventricle and aorta are located midway between the sternum and the top of the mattress on which the patient is lying (Mark 1998, Darovic 2002, White 2003).

Once the mid-chest has been identified, it is good practice to mark it with a marker pen so that anyone else who may be looking after the patient have the same reference point. It is impossible to locate the tip of the catheter exactly with an area on the patient's chest wall. Having said that, the mid-chest is in all probability the area where the catheter tip is located (White 2003). It is more important to be consistent about the pressure measurement taken. For example, where on a particular patient the mid-chest reference point has been identified should be passed on from shift to shift and from clinician to clinician. This essentially ensures that any meaningful changes in the patient's condition can be tracked easily without the shift-to-shift variability that can occur in pressure measurements (Mark 1998).

Zero referencing

The transducer requires a zero reference point as a baseline for all other measurements. Pressure zeroing the transducer eliminates the effect that atmospheric and hydrostatic pressure have on the pressure readings. Atmospheric pressure is the air around us that exerts weight on any object on the Earth's surface and is equal to 760 mmHg (at sea level). The monitor's display is set to read zero, while the transducer stopcock is open and opened to the atmosphere (the process of zeroing the transducer will be explained in detail later in the chapter).

Hydrostatic pressure is the pressure that is exerted on the transducer diaphragm because of its position in relation to the catheter tip. As in atmospheric pressure, the fluid that fills the transducer system also has weight. The force of the fluid's weight, which is applied to the diaphragm in the transducer, is added to the hemodynamic measurement. If a transducer is positioned beneath the tip of the catheter, flow (directed by gravity and the pressure head) is transmitted from the monitor to the diaphragm in the transducer. There is about a 2 mmHg greater measured value for every 1 inch the transducer is below the catheter tip. With the zero reference point and the catheter tip at the same level (vertically), the measurement taken will not be

Quiz 3.2

1. *Do you know why a pressure transducer has to be zeroed?*

2. *Do you know why a pressure transducer has to be leveled?*

affected by hydrostatic pressure (either positive or negative; Mark 1998, Darovic 2002).

The best way to demonstrate this principle is by lowering a bag of intravenous fluid to make sure that the intravenous catheter is patent. If you lower the bag, the negative pressure at the infusion bag means that fluid will flow from the patient to the solution bag from an area of higher pressure to an area of lower pressure, and blood will flow from the patient up the catheter tubing. However, once put back on the drip stand above the level of the intravenous catheter, the positive pressure at the solution bag makes sure that the intravenous infusion will flow from the tubing back into the patient.

Establishing the zero reference point is an important part of monitoring, and should be carried out when the system is set up, at some point during each shift, or if there is question about the reliability of the data being obtained. This is because some of the pressure measurements we make (i.e. pulmonary artery pressure and pulmonary capillary wedge pressure) generate a very narrow range of pressure, and errors in zeroing transducers can make a significant difference to the measurement obtained (Mark 1998).

In order to zero the monitor display, the transducer stopcock must have been leveled to the patients mid-chest first. The stopcock is then closed to the patient and opened to

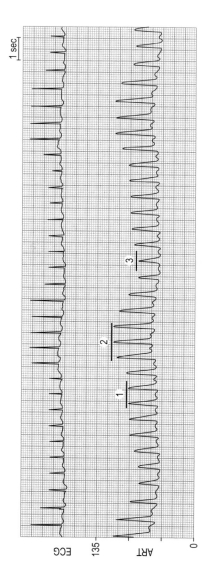

Fig 3.2 Zero referencing. (Reproduced with permission from Mark 1998.)

the atmosphere. The monitored pressure reading should then display a zero value to confirm that the transducer has indeed been zeroed to the atmosphere. The transducer can then either be taped to the patient's thorax at the level of mid-chest, recording pressures with the patient lying on their back, or the pressure transducer can be attached to an intravenous drip stand at mid-chest level, either using a yardstick or a visual assessment. The best way to ensure that the transducer remains at the correct level is to tape the transducer itself to the patient's chest (Darovic 2002).

Over time, drift from the zero reference point occurs. Several factors can cause negative drift. In the case of the transducer domes that have diaphragms (as most do), significant drifts of up to 15 mmHg over a period of 3 hours is possible. If the transducer dome becomes loose, up to 80 mmHg of negative drift can occur. The most common factor that can cause negative drift is the effect of temperature change on the transducer, which can cause a 1–2 mmHg drift for every 10°C change in temperature; this is quite significant. Inaccurate values produced by this drift could result in inappropriate treatments being commenced. This is particularly likely in patients who have low arterial pressures. To prevent this, monitoring systems should be zeroed (Figure 3.2) at least once per shift and at any other point, if the measurements obtained are at all questionable (Darovic 2002).

REFERENCES

Baker D A, Gough D A 1996 Dynamic delay and maximal dynamic error in continuous biosensors. Analytical Chemistry 68: 1292–1297

Barbireri L T; Kaplan A 1983 Artifactual hypotension secondary to intraoperative transducer failure. Anaesthesia Analogues 62: 112–114

Bhatia A, Mackenzie I 2004 Intraoperative hypertensive crisis due to faulty transducer. Anaesthesia 59: 1031–1032

Berne R M, Levy M N 2001 Cardiovascular physiology, 8th edn. Mosby, St Louis, MO

Darovic G O 2002 Hemodynamic monitoring: invasive and non-invasive clinical applications, 3rd edn. Saunders, Philadelphia

D'Orazio P 2003 Biosensors in clinical chemistry. Clinica Chimica Acta 334: 41–69

Gardner R M 1981 Direct blood pressure measurement – dynamic response requirements. Anesthesiology 54: 227–236

Gardner R M, Hollingsworth K W 1986 Optimizing the electrocardiogram and pressure monitoring. Critical Care Medicine 14: 651–658

Lake C L, Hines R L, Blitt C D 2001 Clinical monitoring: practical applications for anaesthesia and critical care. Saunders, Philadelphia

Mark J B 1998 Atlas of cardiovascular monitoring. Churchill Livingstone, Edinburgh

Rolfe B 1990 In vivo chemical sensors for intensive care monitoring. Medical and Biological Engineering and Computing 28: B34–B47

Shinozaki T, Deane R S, Mazuzan J E 1980 The dynamic responses of liquid-filled catheter systems for direct measurements of blood pressure. Anesthesiology 53: 498–504

Tang Z, Louie R F, Kost G J 2002 Principles and performance of point-of-care testing instruments. In: Kost G J (ed.) Principles and practice of point-of-care testing. Lippincott, Williams & Wilkins, Philadelphia: 67–92

Thevenot D R, Toth K, Durst R A et al 2001 Electrochemical biosensors: recommended definitions and classifications. Biosensors and Bioelectronics 16: 121–131

White K 2003 Fast facts for adult critical care. Kathy White Learning Systems, Alabama

SUGGESTED READING

Criner G J, Alonzo E D 1999 Pulmonary pathophysiology. Blackwell Science, Oxford

Gurushanthaiah K, Weinger M B, Englund C E 1995 Visual display format affects the ability of anesthesiologists to detect acute physiologic changes: a laboratory study employing a clinical display simulator. Anesthesiology 83: 1184–1193

Kusumoto F M 1999 Cardiovascular pathophysiology. Blackwell Science, Oxford

Marriott H J L 1968 Practical electrocardiography, 4th edn. Williams & Wilkins, Baltimore

Pearson J E, Gill A, Vadgama P 2000 Analytical aspects of biosensors. Annals of Clinical Biochemistry 37: 119–145

Perloff J K 1987 The clinical recognition of congenital heart disease, 3rd edn. Saunders, Philadelphia

Woods S L, Froelicher E S S, Adams S 2000 Cardiac nursing, 4th edn. Lippincott, Philadelphia

Clinical scenario 1

Margaret Brown is a 70-year-old lady who has been hypertensive since her early 50s. She had an elective repair of her abdominal aortic aneurysm 3 days ago and was then admitted postoperatively to the critical care unit. She is ventilated on pressure-controlled ventilation ($25 \, cmH_2O$) with a positive end-expiratory pressure (PEEP) of $10 \, cmH_2O$. She is sedated and quite comfortable on the ventilator.

You have just taken over her care on the late shift. You were told at handover that she had been hypotensive (95/45) for much of the morning despite a total of 1000 ml in fluid boluses of gelofusin. She has an arterial line in situ. Her central venous pressure (CVP) line is failing to transduce.

- Have this lady's homeostatic mechanisms been triggered?
- How do you know?
- How would you assess the accuracy of the monitoring systems in use?
- How might you optimize the data generated by the monitor?

For answers, see Appendix 2 (page 233).

Interpretation of hemodynamic variables

4 Fundamentals of hemodynamic monitoring

Main objectives

- Explain how to recognize and appreciate the importance of the nurse's role in making an initial assessment of the critically ill patient.
- Highlight the value of less invasive means of obtaining hemodynamic data, while recognizing their limitations, such as ECG monitoring, heart rate and oxygen saturation.
- Provide an understanding of the difference between invasive and non-invasive blood pressure monitoring, and how each can be compromised and optimized.
- Outline the indications for and limitations of central venous cannulation.
- Provide a working knowledge of arterial and CVP waveform morphology.

Introduction

It is important to differentiate between monitoring and measuring. Monitoring is not the same as measuring. Measuring is the intermittent collection of information, repeatedly over time, whereas monitoring is a continuous process. Biological signals are the variables that are monitored and this is done using biomedical sensors. These sensors can be as simple as taking a pulse – your finger senses the impulse and interprets the signal. The use of waveform displays, in addition to digital values, provides important information and detail, patterns of change over time, and trends that would not be possible using intermittent observation (Abrams et al 1989, Mark et al 2000, Darovic 2002).

However simple or complex, in general, all monitoring is affected by many factors that can confuse the interpretation of hemodynamic data. These factors can result in the display of inaccurate or misleading measurements. Sensors have to be able to detect signals accurately. Variables that affect the accuracy of a signal generated, such as physiological, mechanical, electronic or other factors, must be controlled by those who are depending on the measured data for decision-making about the patient. Complex monitoring systems usually incorporate a primary sensing device coupled to a signal amplifier, which then connects to a signal-processing and display device (this has already been covered in detail in a previous section). The user must understand variables influencing each of these components (Mark 1998).

As already stated, monitoring is not therapy and not often diagnostic, essentially because the data do not tell us the cause of the change in a particular measurement. Information from sensors simply assists with the overall assessment of the patient and is taken into consideration alongside

Quiz 4.1

1. *Do you know the difference between measuring and monitoring?*

2. *Can you identify factors that affect the accuracy of data displayed?*

other information contributing to the emerging picture of the patient's condition (O'Rourke et al 1994, Darovic 2002).

A number of factors can result in the display of data that bear no relationship to the patient's hemodynamic status. Such factors include the physical characteristics of fluid-filled monitoring systems, improper zeroing, leveling or the calibration of prepacked monitoring units. In addition, mechanical defects within the monitoring modules and cables, or incorrect positioning or occlusion of the sampling catheter tip can occur. There are also patient-related factors, such as cardiac dysfunction and cyclic pressure effects of spontaneous or mechanical ventilation, which can influence the data (Mark 1998).

The risk–benefit ratio of each and every monitoring system must be appreciated. More invasive monitoring, such as central venous, pulmonary artery or arterial catheters, has to provide sufficiently important new information or therapeutic capability to justify the risk of additional injury to the patient (Figure 4.1).

The nurse is the best monitor

Introduction

In the critical care environment, we are used to having access to hemodynamic monitoring of varying complexity.

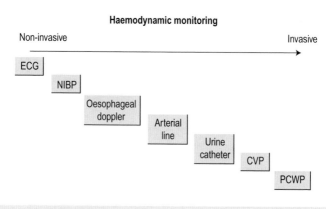

Fig 4.1 Progression of hemodynamic monitoring from non-invasive to invasive.

Having said that, nurses are the best monitors. It is important to have the knowledge and skill to be able to make a quick assessment of a patient without the benefit of equipment. This is particularly important if a patient has just arrived in the critical care unit and has not been connected to hemodynamic monitoring as yet (Smith 2000).

How to make a rapid assessment of a patient's hemodynamic status

The overall assessment of any critically ill patient should be systematic and follow a logical order. It should include the airway (A), breathing (B), circulation (C), deficits (D – neurological) and exposure (E – full-body assessment). There are several courses available to healthcare professionals (Smith 2000) that provide comprehensive and simple methods for approaching not only this assessment, but also the treatment and management of patients. These courses are aimed at nurses and doctors from critical care and ward areas, and are to be recommended. However, the focus of this book is hemodynamic monitoring and we will, therefore, concentrate on this aspect of assessment (Durbin 1990).

When admitting a critically ill patients to the unit, it is important to make a quick and thorough assessment of their cardiovascular stability, in order to make accurate decisions about the priorities for individual patients, and the immediate monitoring and/or treatment they are going to require (Bullock & Colquhoun 2002). Nurses are often the first of the healthcare team to see the patient on the unit and are often relied upon to alert medical staff as to the severity of illness, in particular, a patient's hemodynamic status. Unfortunately, critical illness is often not detected until it has reached an advanced stage and has led to the patients' admission to the critical care unit, making it unlikely to find their cardiovascular systems stable (Smith 2000).

An initial cardiovascular assessment of the patient must begin with the rapid detection and immediate treatment of potential life-threatening situations. Obviously, the earlier potential and actual deteriorations in the condition of patients are recognized (organ impairment or failure), the earlier simple but vital treatments can be initiated (Bullock & Colquhoun 2002).

Simply looking at, listening to and touching patients can reveal a great deal about their cardiovascular stability immediately, and these can be carried out simultaneously. For example, does the patient look pale? Can you see the patient sweating? Are there any visual signs of bleeding? Hemorrhage, visible or not, should be excluded in the surgical patient. Check the contents of any drains, find out when they were last emptied and how much they contained. If the patient is catheterized, check the amount of urine in the bag and find out how much urine they have passed in the last few hours. Oliguria can be a sign of both hypovolemia and a poor cardiac output.

When listening, can the patient talk? Does the patient know where he or she is and what day it is? A reduced conscious level may indicate a poor cardiac output and/or hypovolemia. If patients are able to communicate, find out how they are feeling and what they feel is a problem for them. For example, are they thirsty? This is a good sign that they are centrally dry.

A good start when touching the patient is to feel for peripheral and central pulses. Initially, this allows you to assess their peripheral skin temperature. If their cardiovascular system is compromised, their limbs will be cool and pale, and the capillary refill time will be prolonged. It should be less than 2 seconds (apply pressure to the patient's nail bed for at least 5 seconds before assessment of capillary refill). If the cardiac output is reduced, the peripheries may also be cyanosed and the peripheral veins will look underfilled or even collapsed. The assessment should include checking the presence, strength, rate, regularity and equality of a patient's peripheral and central pulses. A bounding pulse could indicate sepsis, whereas a thready pulse, central or peripheral, may suggest a poor cardiac output (Smith 2000, Bullock & Colquhoun 2002).

Before the person who has transferred the patient to the critical care unit leaves, ensure that you obtain as much information as possible about the patient to enable the critical care team to manage him or her most appropriately. This is a very important point. It is easy to become absorbed in the establishment of monitoring systems and miss vital information being handed over. A detailed history, present and past, should be provided, including the events leading up to this and any previous admissions to critical care. It should be clear which medical team have responsibility for the patient so that liaison can take place between teams without delay. Most of all, the handing over of all relevant and up-to-date documentation is vital, including the dynamics and contact details of family members together with their understanding of the current situation (Smith 2000).

Early interventions

Having made a rapid overall assessment of the patient's hemodynamic status, it is important to start to respond immediately while monitoring is being established and the accuracy of the data materializing is being optimized.

The priorities will obviously vary with each individual patient, but they are likely to be related to the patient's fluid management, control of any obvious hemorrhage and the provision of adequate tissue perfusion. How quickly this can be achieved will depend on where the patient has been transferred from. For example, in the trauma patient from the accident and emergency department, the patient is likely to have been receiving oxygen therapy and have adequate venous access (two 16G peripheral lines, and perhaps a central and arterial line). If this is not the case, giving adequate amounts of oxygen, obtaining venous and arterial access and giving intravenous fluids would be major priorities.

Oxygen therapy

It is crucial to give high oxygen concentrations to all patients who have become critically ill regardless of the cause. It should also be remembered that, in the critically ill patients, the risks associated with giving inadequate oxygen therapy far out way those associated with giving too high a concentration, regardless of any pre-existing pulmonary disease. Clinically, the effects of oxygen therapy can be assessed by noting the patients' color, respiratory pattern, and their rate and use of accessory muscles for breathing. These observations can be corroborated once arterial access has been established and arterial blood gases analysed. These results can then be used to guide further therapy (Smith 2000, Bullock & Colquhoun 2001).

Intravenous fluids

If the patient is hypotensive, the administration of intravenous fluids should be a priority while the underlying cause is being investigated. Having said that, establishing whether the cause of the hypotension is due to a reduction in cardiac output or a change in systemic vascular resistance is important. The management of hypotension with fluid therapy will depend on the individual patient. For example, the surgical patient is likely to be hypotensive because of excessive blood loss (during the procedure or as an ongoing problem) and fluid replacement volumes may need to be high. However, in a patient with known cardiac failure or following an acute cardiac event, fluid therapy is likely to be less aggressive and the response assessed frequently (e.g. evidence of pulmonary edema). The aim of giving any fluid bolus is to increase the circulatory volume and renal perfusion. Having said that, identifying which patients will respond to fluid challenges can be difficult (we will return to this in a later chapter). It should be remembered that, if a patient is going to respond to a fluid bolus, that response is fairly immediate. Waiting half an hour or more simply wastes time in the administration of further appropriate therapies (e.g. if the patient appears to be adequately fluid loaded and yet a reduced urine output persists; Smith 2000).

It should be remembered that hypotension is a late sign of cardiovascular compromise and is a sign that the body is failing to maintain homeostasis through its usual mechanisms (e.g. an increase in pulse rate and vasoconstriction). Untreated, this can result in poor perfusion to the major organs (brain, heart and kidneys), the signs of which will appear as, for example, altered conscious level, hypotension and oliguria, if they are not already present.

Any reduction in the flow of blood to the brain (autoregulated within a specific range of 60–140 mmHg) will lead to changes in the ability of patients to maintain consciousness (drowsiness or coma), and their awareness and ability to make rationale decisions about what is happening to them (confusion, irritation). The flow of blood to the coronary circulation depends on the diastolic blood pressure. If the blood pressure decreases and the heart rate increases, the filling time will be reduced and may compromise the perfusion of the coronary blood vessels. The normal functioning of the kidneys depends on adequate blood flow and pressure. Underperfusion of the kidneys is the most common cause of acute tubular necrosis and can be avoided by responding rapidly to inadequate urine output (less than 0.5 ml/kg per hour for two consecutive hours; Smith, 2000). Obviously, the bladder should be palpated to exclude acute retention and the patency of a urine catheter should be established before responding with any treatment (Smith 2000, Bullock & Coquhoun 2001).

ECG monitoring

The electrocardiogram (ECG) is probably the most basic hemodynamic monitoring we undertake (Figure 4.2). Having said that, it is an extremely important variable to monitor and is vital when looking at the other

Fig 4.2 Multiple-channel recording of ECG lead II, arterial blood pressure (ABP) and central venous pressure (CVP). The a-, c- and v-waves in the CVP trace are identified by their location in the diastolic (a-wave) or systolic (c- and v-waves) portion of the cardiac cycle. (Reproduced with permission from Mark 1998.)

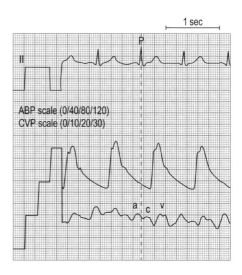

ABP scale (0/40/80/120)
CVP scale (0/10/20/30)

hemodynamic monitoring that is carried out. This is especially true when analysing waveforms obtained from other signals. The ability to analyse abnormal cardiac rhythms accurately requires a great deal of expertise and experience. In-depth ECG interpretation is outside the scope of this book and there are many excellent texts dedicated to the subject (Thaler 2003). However, it is worth outlining the basic principles of how to obtain an optimal ECG signal and how to recognize when the rhythm is not normal at least.

Anything you can do to improve the electrical contact with the patients skin is going to optimize the signal obtained. For example, adhesive electrodes should be attached to the patient's chest after the skin has been cleaned with alcohol. This causes the skin's natural oil to dissolve (Darovic 2002). The gel in the center of the electrode enhances the electrical contact and care should be taken not to remove this. If the patient to be monitored has any body hair where the electrodes are going to be positioned, this should be shaved.

There are some basic principles that can be applied to any ECG trace in order to achieve an optimal signal that are advocated by the Resuscitation Council (Bullock & Colquhoun 2002). Firstly, can you identify any electrical activity (i.e. are there any positive or negative deflections from the baseline)? (A totally flat line is likely to be because an ECG lead has come off.) Secondly, what is the rate of ventricular contractions? (Is the rate greater that 60 beats/minute and less than 100 beats/minute?) Thirdly, is the rhythm regular or not? (Is the gap between each complex consistent?) And how wide are the QRS complexes? (They should be less than three small squares.) Finally, are the atria contracting (can you see any P-waves)? If you can, how are they related to that of the ventricular contractions? (Is the gap between them normal and do they follow each other consistently?)

Heart rate

Monitoring and estimating the heart rate has to be the most common component of ECG monitoring. Having said that, it is also often taken for granted. The ability to estimate the heart rate rapidly by looking at the monitor's ECG trace provides useful information to help us to make quick decisions about the patient's hemodynamic status (Seeley 2000).

The majority of current monitors have the facility to look at several ECG leads at one time in order to detect electrical activity. The main aim of this is to detect the R-wave, which allows the monitor to calculate the heart rate properly and accurately, without being affected by a single noisy lead, or one in which the R-waves are difficult to identify (low amplitude). The QRS complex is used as an identified starting point for measurement of the heart rate. Having said that, how the signal is subsequently processed will vary from monitor to monitor. This can then affect the monitor's ability to reflect transient changes in heart rate in the digital value displayed. The displayed digital values for the heart rate that appear on the monitor are derived from an algorithm (Mark 1998). This algorithm generates an average (over a period of beats) and then displays a number. Generally the number is updated every 5–12 seconds, depending on the individual monitor. Depending on what algorithm is being used by the monitor, only a slight change in heart rate is displayed in the case of a short run of an arrhythmia. Potentially, this can then be missed by the person doing the monitoring. As for all pressure monitoring, generally, the heart rate displayed on a monitor is generated by the use of an average filter. You may think that to be truly accurate the reading displayed should be beat to beat. However, because the R–R interval naturally varies, the display would be flashing all the time. Whatever the type of algorithm that is being used by the monitor, accuracy must be confirmed by looking at the ECG in order to confirm the digital value for heart rate. In order to pick up transient changes in heart rate, it is useful to look periodically at the monitor's ECG history screen. This screen, which appears on most current monitors, may show an event that was not seen at the time and did not trigger an alarm (Wilkinson et al 2000, Darovic 2002).

The display of inaccurate heart rates by the monitor occurs when the ECG trace is affected by electrical interference, such as other monitoring or supportive equipment, or by the patient moving, for example, from muscle twitching. If a patient is being paced, it can cause problems for monitors to calculate an accurate heart rate. For example, the presence of tall pacing spikes and, classically, high amplitude can cause miscalculation of the heart rate because the monitor has interpreted them as R-waves. This is also true if the patient has tall T-waves and the monitor fails to differentiate between the two. The best way to manage this is by using a range of techniques. For example, decreasing the ECG gain (the amount of amplification applied to the signal). It increases or decreases the actual signal, not the volume. Also, adjusting the sensitivity of R-wave detection, or changing the ECG lead to one that has a smaller pacing spike or reduced T-wave. If the patient is being temporarily paced, try changing from unipolar to bipolar pacing, which will alter the amplitude of the pacing spike (Mark 1998, Hope et al 2003).

Either the arterial trace (if the patient has invasive arterial pressure monitoring in progress) or plethysmograph of the pulse oximeter should also be taken into consideration when differentiating between real and spurious readings. In order to restore a good trace, you should check the attachment of the electrodes (see 'ECG monitoring') or alter the signal filter, which will remove artifact (other signals that affect the one being monitored). There are several ways you can estimate what would be the real heart rate for any 1 minute. However, in the case of an irregular heart rate, they are not very accurate (Bullock & Colquhoun 2002).

Monitoring the pulse rate and heart rate at the same time can be useful, and is the usual practice. The heart rate is taken from the ECG trace. The pulse trace can be obtained from the pulse oximeter or invasive arterial blood pressure waveform. Unless the patient is peripherally shut down or has significant arterial occlusive disease, the plethysmograph trace can be used for pulse measurement (Mark 1998, Hope et al 2003).

Oxygen saturation

The oxygen saturation level (SaO_2) is a measurement of the amount of oxygen that is bound to hemoglobin (oxyhemoglobin). This is in contrast to the partial pressure of oxygen, which is the amount of oxygen dissolved in arterial blood. Pulse oximetry makes use of a spectrophotometer in order to determine the amount of light that is absorbed by the hemoglobin in a patient's arterial blood. The pulse oximeter probe passes a red and near-infrared light of two different wavelengths through the appendage it is attached to (i.e. toe, finger or ear) and compares the level of light transmission (Smith 2000, Grap 2002).

Pulse oximeters (and other monitors for that matter) display a time-weighted average. This means that the number displayed on the monitor is the average saturation of oxygen over the previous 8–12 seconds. It is reassuring to see a normal saturation of oxygen but it needs to be clear that, when it drops, the patient's SaO_2 actually dropped some 8–12 seconds ago (Darovic 2002). Adequate perfusion of the tissue is necessary for an accurate reading and conditions that reduce perfusion affect the reading. For example, hypothermia, hypotension and some drugs that can cause peripheral vasoconstriction can result in false low readings (Bullock & Colquhoun 2002). The SaO_2 can vary with the partial pressure of oxygen, body temperature and the actual structure of hemoglobin. On average, the oxygen saturation should be 96–100% and does not follow the partial pressure of oxygen proportionately (Sequin et al 2000, Van de Louw et al 2001). Procedural tips for pulse oximetry are shown in Box 4.1.

The acidity or alkalinity (pH) of the blood can affect the ability of oxygen to bind to hemoglobin. From the oxygen dissociation curve (see Figure 2.2), you can see the changes that take place in the oxygen binding to and release from hemoglobin with the pH of the blood. With a pH of less than 7.35 (acidic), the oxygen dissociation curve shifts to the left with a lower oxygen saturation, higher release of

---

Box 4.1 How to get the most out of pulse oximetry monitoring.
(Reproduced with permission from Darovic 2002)

1. Inspect the sensor and cable for defects before application.
2. Choose a warm sampling site with good capillary refill. If the patient is intensely vasoconstricted or has peripheral vascular disease, use a nasal or earlobe sensor. Avoid application of the sensor to areas of edema, or sites distal to an arterial line or automated blood pressure cuff.
3. Cleanse the intended monitoring site with alcohol.
4. Remove acrylic nails, and black, blue, green, metallic or thickly applied nail polish. Long fingernails prevent correct positioning of the finger under the diodes (inflexible probes).
5. Make sure that the light-emitting and light-receiving sensors are oppositely aligned.
6. Following use, cleanse the sensor and cable with disinfectant (hospital protocol).

---

oxygen and a reduced oxygen binding. On the other hand, if the blood pH is greater than 7.45 (alkalotic), the oxyhemoglobin desaturation curve shifts to the right with a higher saturation of oxygen, higher oxygen binding and lower oxygen release (Darovic 2002). The saturation of oxygen is also affected by temperature changes and the level of carbon dioxide in the blood.

Non-invasive blood pressure monitoring

Blood flows through the arteries under force and blood pressure is a measure of this force on the arterial walls contained within the arterial system. Blood flow and pressure are pulsatile, representing systolic and diastolic activity. Arterial blood pressure has both numerical and non-numerical components. The numerical components comprise systolic, diastolic, mean and pulse pressures. The non-numerical components are the shape or morphology of the waveform, and the variations that occur during respiration. Non-invasive blood pressure monitoring generally only provides us with numerical values. However, newer methods provide waveforms (Durbin 1990, Gravlee & Brockschmidt 1990, Geddes 1991).

Non-invasive monitoring of the cardiovascular system has been considered an important part of patient management for thousands of years, starting with the noting of the nature (quality, regularity) of the peripheral pulses. This information was then used to predict time of death (Durbin 1990). However, the pulsatile nature of circulating blood (blood pressure) and its subsequent measurement did not occur until 1733. Early measurements were taken invasively using animals. The first hydraulic cuff was used to occlude a peripheral artery as it passed over a bony prominence. The systolic pressure was measured by reducing the cuff pressure until the hydraulic system detected the pulsations. It was Riva-Rocci (1887) who first measured blood pressure using a cuff inflated with air. However, in 1905, it was Korotkoff who proposed the concept of using auscultatory methods to obtain systolic and diastolic measurements (Korotkoff 1905). This remains a standard method of non-invasive measurement of blood pressure today (Durbin 1990, McAlister & Straus 2001).

There are basically three techniques for measuring the blood pressure non-invasively (Durbin 1990, O'Brien et al 2001). Some of these are manual methods and some are automatic. Both the use of an occlusive cuff to detect flow distal to it or oscillations in a cuff that is pressurized (e.g. Riva-Rocci, Dinamap) can be achieved either by palpation or auscultatory methods (Ramsey 1994, Young et al 1995). 'Arterial plethysmomanometry' from a cuff that is partially pressurized provides beat-by-beat monitoring. The Tensymeter (TL-100; Tensys Medical Inc. 2003) is a relatively new method of measuring radial arterial blood pressure continuously utilizing a transdermal pressure sensor. Both the average pressure and pulse pressure measured by the transducer rise as the transducer compresses against the skin. Once the artery has been sensed, the compression motor moves over the radial artery (sliding motion) until the optimal signal is located. Subsequently, the externally sensed pressure is transduced as a waveform that appears on the monitor. This waveform closely resembles the arterial pressure waveform that would be obtained from an intra-arterial line (Tensys Medical Inc. 2003).

Detecting blood pressure (both systolic and diastolic) manually is classically by the identification of the Korotkoff sounds (Korotkoff 1905), otherwise known as the Riva-Rocci method (after the person who was given credit for proposing it). Ordinarily, blood flows through major arteries with very little turbulence (because of their smooth inner lining) and cannot be heard through a stethoscope. However, if the artery is compressed by an inflated cuff, vibrations and sounds that have a low frequency can be detected (Korotkoff sounds). The systolic point is noted as the sounds start and flow begins. The diastolic point is noted when these sounds become less clear and then disappear as the partially occluded artery has its flow returned (Ostchega et al 2003).

The accuracy of this method of blood pressure determination is dependent on several factors. For example, the cuff should be the correct size for the individual patient. A cuff that is too small, has been applied too loosely or has air in it before the measurement is taken will give falsely high readings. A cuff that is too large will give a falsely low reading. Having said that, the degree of error is greatest if the cuff is too small (Iyriboz et al 1994). The correct cuff width is dependent on the diameter of the limb used to take the measurement. As a general guide, the cuff length should be at least 80% of the circumference of the limb used and 40% of the limb's width (Mark 1998, Darovic 2002).

Automated devices have simplified and standardized the measurement of blood pressure, but the method of blood pressure measurement using these devices is different from the traditional auscultation method and can lead to misinterpretation. Quite simply, the automated cuff inflates and deflates automatically, detecting the presence of the amplitude of pulsations in the arm. The peak amplitude is the mean arterial pressure, and the systolic and diastolic pressures are then calculated from an analysis of the peak amplitude of pulsations and the rate of increase and decline of its pulsations. Therefore, the mean arterial pressure is a measured value, and the systolic and diastolic readings are only calculated values. This is why, when compared to an invasive systolic and diastolic blood pressure measured from an arterial line, there will be a discrepancy, because invasive pressure monitoring does the opposite. It directly measures the systolic and diastolic pressures, and calculates the mean from those measurements. In patients with cardiovascular insufficiency for whatever reason (e.g. shock), the Korotkoff sounds may be difficult to identify. This is because the change in sound frequency (generally associated with a fall in blood pressure) makes it difficult to detect them with normal hearing ability. This inability to identify Korotkoff sounds is a result of either poor stroke volume or vasoconstriction, or both, whatever the underlying cause (Pauca et al 2001, Darovic 2002).

Although invasive measurement of arterial blood pressure is more costly, has the potential for more complications, and requires more technical expertise to initiate and maintain, it is more appropriate in critically ill patients because it is known to be more accurate (assuming the transducer

Quiz 4.2

1. Do you know which is the most important measure: systolic, diastolic or mean?

2. Can you identify the patient and technical factors that affect the accuracy of non-invasive blood pressure readings?

Quiz 4.3

1. If the pressure transducer is raised above the level of the heart, will the pressure reading be higher or lower than it would be if it were level with the heart?

2. What are the most common mistakes made with pressure monitoring?

set has been prepared, connected, leveled and zeroed correctly) than non-invasive methods (Figure 4.3). In addition, it provides us with continuous measurements, as they exist in the patient on a beat-by-beat basis (Wilkinson et al 2000, Millasseau et al 2003, O'Rourke 2003).

Invasive blood pressure monitoring

When compared with intermittent monitoring of the arterial blood pressure, the continuous monitoring of arterial blood pressure allows the detection of moment-to-moment pressure changes. Having said that, even invasive measurement of arterial blood pressure is frequently interrupted by electrical and mechanical distortions, and interference (artifact), line sampling and flushing. Surprisingly, this has been shown to affect arterial trace availability for up to 15% of

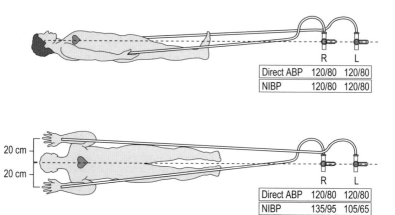

Fig 4.3 Invasive direct arterial blood pressure (ABP) compared to non-invasive indirect blood pressure (NIBP) in the supine (top) and lateral (bottom) positions. In this example, direct arterial blood pressure measured from both right and left radial arteries, and non-invasive blood pressure measured from both arms all record the same value for blood pressure with the patient in the supine position. When the patient assumes the right lateral position, both right and left pressure transducers remain at the level of the heart and record the same direct arterial blood pressure. However, the left arm is now located 20 cm above the heart and the non-invasive blood pressure recorded from this arm will be lower, while the non-invasive blood pressure recorded from the right arm located 20 cm below the heart will be higher. (Reproduced with permission from Mark 1998.)

the time (Mark 1998, Smulyan et al 2001). Interference from the external arterial line component does increase the systolic blood pressure reading and lower the diastolic blood pressure reading. However, the mean arterial pressure is unaffected. Patient-related factors, such as their own cardiovascular system, can also create interference. Generally, this occurs when patients are either hypertensive or tachycardic, have small peripheral blood vessels, as a result of old age, or have some form of cardiovascular disease, such as atherosclerosis (Durbin 1990, Mitchell et al 2003, O'Rourke 2003, White 2003).

The evidence supporting accuracy, either good or bad, between invasive and non-invasive blood pressure measurements is inconsistent, making it sensible to establish individual principles to follow in practice. Values for non-invasive systolic pressure are equal to or slightly higher than invasive systolic pressure values (in normotensive patients). In patients with high blood pressure, non-invasive methods provide lower values than invasive methods for systolic pressure. Conversely, in hypotension, non-invasive methods give slightly higher readings for systolic pressure than invasive methods (O'Rourke 2003). Interpretation of mean arterial pressure values is dependent on the method used to calculate it. In general, non-invasive measurement of the mean arterial pressure provides values that are equal to or slightly higher than those taken using invasive measurement. When diastolic arterial pressure is measured by non-invasive means, it is generally slightly higher than when measured invasively (Mark 1998, London et al 2001, Darovic 2002).

The causes of disagreement between invasive and non-invasive blood pressure measurement are summarized in Boxes 4.2 and 4.3.

When questioning the accuracy of invasive blood pressure readings, it is fair to say that, on the whole, a non-invasive blood pressure is then taken and the two compared. Having said that, it should not be a surprise to find a natural discrepancy between the two readings, because they are measuring different things (see 'Non-invasive blood pressure monitoring' for more detail). Invasive blood pressure measurement is just that – a pressure – whereas non-invasive blood pressure measurement is a flow measurement

---

Quiz 4.4

1. *What are the components of the invasive arterial blood pressure waveform?*

2. *Can you outline what the true mean arterial pressure is?*

Box 4.2 Patient-related factors that cause disagreement between direct and indirect blood pressure measurements. (Reproduced with permission from Mark 1998)

Regional arterial pressure gradients
- Atherosclerosis
- Peripheral vascular disease
- Aortic dissection
- Arterial embolism
- Surgical retractors
- Patient position

Generalized arterial pressure gradients
- Severe vasoconstriction and shock
- Peripheral vasodilation with rewarming after cardiopulmonary bypass
- Normal peripheral pulse pressure widening

Box 4.3 Technical factors that can cause disagreement between direct and indirect blood pressure measurements. (Reproduced with permission from Mark 1998)

Cuff problems
- Size too small leads to overestimation
- Fit in a conical-shaped arm
- Extrinsic cuff compression
- Limb position relative to heart
- Rapid deflation leads to underestimation

Physiologic problems and method limitations
- Rapid pressure changes
- Dysrhythmias
- Severe vasoconstriction and shock
- Shivering and patient movement
- Beat-to-beat variation (e.g. pulsus alternans)

beyond an air-filled cuff. An alternative method of comparing invasive and non-invasive measurements is by using the 'return to flow' method. This simply involves the identification of a pulse, distal to a blood-pressure cuff. The pulse can be detected with a finger, Doppler flow detector, pulse oximeter or an invasive arterial line. Systolic pressure is then established by inflating and deflating the cuff, using the point at which the pulse is first detected on deflation as the systolic pressure. This is then compared to the systolic blood pressure reading taken from the invasive arterial waveform (Durbin 1990).

The commencement of any invasive monitoring should be justified in terms of the cost and benefit to the patient. If frequent sampling of blood is required, then the need for arterial cannulation is justified. In addition, under some situations, the blood pressure cannot be detected by indirect methods (e.g. cardiovascular shock or systemic vasoconstriction). In these situations, although it may not be possible to obtain a non-invasive blood pressure reading, the insertion of an arterial line and transducing of an accurate waveform, may well demonstrate that the patient actually has a normal or even a high blood pressure. The most important reason to monitor arterial blood pressure directly is because of the information about the patient's diagnosis that it can provide, often by simply looking at the arterial waveform itself (Mark 1998, Darovic 2002).

Quiz 4.5

1. Can you identify the indicators for invasive arterial pressure monitoring?

2. Why do invasive and non-invasive blood pressures yield different numbers?

Components of the arterial waveform

The flow of blood from the left ventricle into the arterial system, following ejection, creates a wave of pressure. This pressure is then conveyed to the peripheral arterial system. The transmission of the pressure wave occurs much more rapidly than the flow of blood. This is an important point. When the radial pulse is detected by the finger, what is being felt is the wave of pressure being transmitted through the arterial system, not the blood flow that has just been ejected from the left ventricle. This flow arrives at the same point (in the radial artery) a few beats afterwards because the wave of pressure travels much faster than blood flow. The rate of blood flow is 0.5 m/s compared to 10 m/s for the pressure wave (Mark 1998; Pauca et al 2001; Weber et al 2004).

For ease of description, the arterial waveform can be divided into two components, systole and diastole. During systole, blood is ejected into the aorta from the left ventricle, followed by peripheral arterial runoff during diastole. The systolic components of the arterial pressure waveform follow the R-wave of the ECG. It is worth remembering that the waveform generated as a result of these events is simply a graphical representation of changes in systemic arterial pressure that take place during each phase. The arterial pressure waveform consists of a steep rise in pressure, the upstroke, a peak of pressure, followed by a fall in pressure and decline (Figure 4.4). These rises and falls in pressure correspond to the period of left ventricular systolic ejection (Mark 1998).

Aortic valve closure at the end of diastole is marked by a dicrotic notch, which graphically separates systole from diastole. It appears on the downslope of the arterial blood pressure waveform. The position in the arterial system at

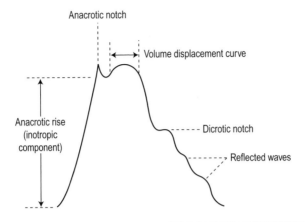

Anacrotic notch

Volume displacement curve

Anacrotic rise
(inotropic
component)

Dicrotic notch

Reflected waves

Fig 4.4 The arterial pressure/pulse pressure wave. (Reproduced with permission from Darovic 2002.)

Quiz 4.6

1. *Do you know what the dicrotic notch is?*

2. *Can you explain how it differs when recorded from the aorta and the radial artery?*

which the waveform is being transduced affects how clearly it can be seen (Figure 4.5). For example, if it is viewed from the central aorta, it is clearly defined and reflects aortic valve closure, and can thus be useful as a marker. However, if it is transduced from further down the arterial system, say from the radial artery, it is affected by the properties of the arterial wall and is less clearly defined (smoother), and aortic valve closure can only be estimated. During diastole, the arterial blood pressure decreases gradually, reaching its lowest point at the end of diastole. On the ECG, this gradual decline in pressure follows the T-wave (Hope et al 2003, White 2003).

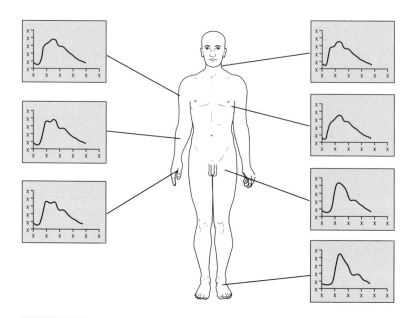

Fig 4.5 Contour of the arterial pressure waveform relative to the site used for pressure measurement. (Reproduced from Wilson R F 1992 Cardiovascular physiology. In: Critical care manual. Davis, Philadelphia.)

Both the systolic and the diastolic components of the arterial blood pressure waveform are fairly easy to identify. Having said that, their relation to the ECG waveform requires more consideration. The systolic upstroke of the radial artery pressure trace does not appear for 120–180 ms after the R-wave (Mark 1998). Therefore, when using the arterial pressure wave as a guide to the timing of cardiac events, it is important to bear these delays in mind. They occur for a number of reasons (Mark 1998, Darovic 2002, Millasseau et al 2003):

- the process of electrical depolarization;
- isovolumetric contraction;
- the opening of the aortic valve;
- ejection from the left ventricle and the subsequent transmission of the pressure wave, not only from the aorta to

the radial artery, but also the pressure signal from there to the pressure transducer.

Mean arterial pressure

Throughout the cardiac cycle, blood is being forced under pressure around the arterial system. The average of this force is the mean arterial pressure. It is a useful measure because it is the same throughout the arterial system and is not affected by monitor factors, such as artifact, dampening or frequency response. In addition, the measure itself can be used to calculate the systemic vascular resistance, and also is similar to the pressure both within the systemic circulations and cerebral capillary bed (Mark 1998).

The accuracy of the mean arterial pressure depends on how it has been arrived at. The midpoint between the systolic and diastolic pressure is known as the arithmetic mean. It is arrived at by assuming that, at 60 beats/min, for example, diastole will be two-thirds of the total cardiac cycle. In reality, this is not the case because heart rates are variable. In practice, the mean arterial blood pressure is often estimated as diastolic pressure plus one-third times the pulse pressure. This can be misleading because the height and width of the waveform affect the mean arterial pressure generated. For example, falsely low mean arterial pressure readings can result from the interpretation of a narrow or thin waveform (these spend more time reading lower pressures). In contrast, wide or full waveforms can result in falsely high mean arterial pressures (these spend more time reading higher pressures).

A mean arterial pressure that has been derived by invasive means can be relied upon to be accurate. This is because the monitored and displayed values for systolic and diastole pressure are taken from the peak (systolic) and trough (diastolic) pressures. The area under the arterial waveform curve is averaged over several beats. Mean arterial pressure is equal to the area under the curve divided by the beat period (Mark 1998, Wilkinson et al 2000, Darovic 2002).

The use of consistent scales when monitoring arterial pressure is important to enable a quick estimation of both systolic and diastolic pressures by a simple glance, without having to rely on the numeric display (Mark 1998, Darovic 2002).

The various components of the arterial pressure wave can be reproduced fairly accurately by creating two sine waves, even though these pressure waves have been detected from different sites in the body, affecting the waveform shape. The effects of gravity on the flow of blood affects arterial pressure by increasing it as blood flows downwards from the heart, and decreasing it as the blood flows upwards from the level of the heart.

Changes in the arterial wave as it moves from the aorta to the periphery occur. These changes are characteristic. The upstroke of the arterial waveform is sharper and the systolic peak is higher. The appearance of the dicrotic notch is later and the diastolic pressure wave is more distinctive. The end-diastolic pressure is also lower (Mark 1998). When compared to central aortic pressure in waveforms transduced

Quiz 4.7

1. *Do you know why consistent scales are important in arterial pressure monitoring?*

2. *Can you explain the delays that occur between the ECG and arterial waveform?*

Quiz 4.8

1. *Do you know how the arterial waveform is reproduced?*
2. *Do you know what the pressure difference is between the aorta and the radial artery?*

from a peripheral site, the systolic pressure will be higher and the diastolic pressure lower. This results in a wider pulse pressure. Despite these differences, there is little significant change in mean arterial pressure (slightly higher) from a peripheral site when compared with the central aorta (London et al 2001, Darovic 2002, White 2003).

Central venous pressure

The measurement of the central venous pressure (CVP), after the heart rate and arterial blood pressure, is the most common variable that is monitored in the critically ill patient and is generally used to guide fluid therapy. The reason for this is that the amount of pressure generated in the atria during its contraction is thought to not only reflect left atrial filling but also to reflect preload of the heart. This is based on the assumption that the left and right atria distend to the same degree, but also that the pressure generated during that distension equates to volume (Merrer et al 2001).

When the central venous pressure is transduced via an unobstructed fluid-filled system (as described previously) to a monitor and amplifier, a waveform and digital value is displayed. Obviously, the accuracy of the display depends on the central venous catheter being in the correct position. In addition, it is worth remembering that the digital value displayed on the monitor is generally the mean central venous pressure, not taken from the peak of the a-wave, which is the pressure of interest (Mark 1995, McGee & Gould 2003). Having said that, the range of pressures generated by atrial contraction is small and it is probably clinically insignificant (Darovic 2002).

The central venous pressure and right atrial pressure (RAP) generate similar pressure waveforms and the terms are frequently used interchangeably. Central venous pressure is usually recorded from either a catheter with its tip positioned in the superior vena cava or from a pulmonary artery catheter's proximal (right atrial) lumen. When examining the central venous pressure waveform, it can be seen to consist of five phasic events (Figure 4.6 and Table 4.1).

There are three pressure peaks (a, c and v) and two pressure descents (x, y). The first deflection is the a-wave and occurs at end-diastole, created by contraction of the atrium increasing atrial pressure, assisting the filling of the ventricle through the tricuspid value. On the ECG, it follows the P-wave. Following the a-wave, atrial pressure starts to fall smoothly as the atrium relaxes. The next pressure increase is the c-wave generated by the start of ventricular systole. This wave is a brief increase in atrial pressure as a result of isovolumetric ventricular contraction closing the tricuspid

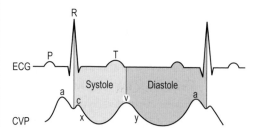

Fig 4.6 A normal central venous pressure (CVP) waveform with its three systolic components (c-wave, x-descent, v-wave) and two diastolic components (y-descent, a-wave). (Reproduced with permission from Mark 1998.)

Table 4.1 Normal central venous pressure. (Reproduced with permission from Mark 1998)

Waveform component	Phase of cardiac cycle	Mechanical event
a-wave	End-diastole	Atrial contraction
c-wave	Early systole	Isovolumetric ventricular contraction, tricuspid motion toward right atrium
v-wave	Late systole	Systolic filling of atrium
x-descent	Mid-systole	Atrial relaxation, descent of the base, systolic collapse
y-descent	Early diastole	Early ventricular filling, diastolic collapse

valve and causing it to bulge towards the atrium. On the ECG, the c-wave follows the R-wave.

The geometry of the atria is affected by the contraction of the ventricles and ejection of blood. This and atrial contraction causes atrial pressure to fall during ventricular systole. This fall in atrial pressure is the x-descent. The v-wave, which is the final pressure peak, is caused by the filling of the atrium during the latter part of systole, while the tricuspid valve is still closed. On the ECG, the v-wave reaches its maximum pressure just after the T-wave. The pressure in the atrium then falls (y-descent), as the tricuspid valve opens and blood flows from the atrium to the ventricle (Mark 1998, Amar et al 2001, Darovic 2002).

The use of the peak of the R-wave as a reference point on the ECG is a valuable aid to the interpretation of any waveforms. This is otherwise known as the 'Z' point. Although it could be argued that it is not an exact marker of the end of diastole and beginning of systole, it is an easily recognized reference point. The atrial pressure waveform has three systolic components (c-wave, x-descent and v-wave) and two diastolic components (y-descent, a-wave) in relation to the cardiac cycle and the mechanical ventricular events. It is essential to remember the chemical, electrical and mechanical events that generate the pressure peaks and troughs, and to use the ECG trace, particularly the ECG R-wave to differentiate between the end of diastole and start of systole (Mark 1998, Darovic 2002).

It is better to use the ECG in order to interpret the CVP waveform rather than the arterial waveform. This is because several events contribute to a delay in the appearance of the arterial blood pressure waveform, which can amount to 200 ms, between the radial arterial pressure rise (anacrotic rise) and the R-wave on the ECG (see Figure 4.6). This sequence of events (delays) results in the delayed appearance of the anacrotic rise in relation to the c-wave. Although atrial pressure peaks are known as systolic (c, v) or diastolic (a) waves, according to where they begin in relation to the cardiac cycle, they are generally identified according to their location, not their onset or upstroke. It is easiest to think of the v-wave as a systolic wave (Mark 1998, Darovic 2002).

The atrial pressure trace is usually recognized by three atrial pressure peaks (a, c, v) and two troughs (x, y). Having said that, abnormalities in the heart rate can affect this. In bradycardic patients, each component of the atrial pressure trace becomes easier to identify. For example, diastole is elongated and it may be possible to identify an additional plateau pressure, known as the h-wave, during the middle or later part of diastole. In tachycardic patients, the opposite occurs and the atrial pressure waves can merge, resulting in the a–c-wave appearing as one pressure rise. The x- and y-pressure falls are shorter. Overall, this makes the waveform more difficult to interpret (Mark 1998, Darovic 2002).

Ordinarily, the mean pressure in the left atria is higher than mean pressure in the right atria. Having said that, in some patients, this normal pressure gradient reverses briefly during the cardiac cycle, usually during contraction of the atria (a-wave). If the foramen ovale is patent, there is a potential risk of materials such as blood clots and gas passing through it (Mark 1998, Darovic 2002).

The shape and nature of the waveforms generated by both the left and right atrial pressures are minimal. However, some differences can be identified. Because depolarization of the right atria begins in the sinoatrial node, which is also located on the right side of the heart (superior vena cava/right atria), the a-wave appears slightly earlier on the right atrial pressure waveform than that on the left (the a- and c-waves seen in the waveform generated by the right atrial pressure are generally separate). In addition, the a-wave on the right is more defined, which suggests that atrial contraction on the right side of the heart is more forceful than the left, resulting in a smaller increase in the size of the left atria during the passive phase of the cardiac cycle. An interval exists between right atria and right ventricular contraction, resulting in a more prominent v-wave in the normal left atrial waveform. There is also an interval between left atrial and ventricular contraction, which is greater by approximately 40 ms (Mark 1998, Darovic 2002).

In order to interpret the central venous pressure waveform accurately in relation to the cardiac cycle (using the ECG trace), it is essential to use a two-channel recorder to print off a section of these two waveforms. Only then can the rises and falls in atrial pressure be analysed and interpreted, as a result of the chemical and electrical events with which they coincide during the cardiac cycle.

REFERENCES

Abrams J H, Cerra F, Holcroft J W 1989 Cardiopulmonary monitioring. In: Wilmore D W, Brennan M F, Harken A H, et al (eds) Care of the surgical patient 1: critical care. Scientific American Medicine, New York: 1–27

Amar D, Melendez J A, Zhang H, Dobres C, Leung D H Y, Padilla R E 2001 Correlation of peripheral venous pressure and central venous pressure in surgical patients. Journal of Cardiothoracic and Vascular Anesthesia 15: 40–43.

Bullock I, Colquhoun M 2002 ALS manual. Resuscitation Council, London

Darovic G O 2002 Hemodynamic monitoring: invasive and noninvasive clinical applications 3rd edn. Saunders, Philadelphia

Durbin C G 1990 Noninvasive hemodynamic monitoring. Respiratory Care 7: 709–717

Gardner R M 1981 Direct blood pressure measurement – dynamic response requirements. Anesthesiology 54: 227–236

Geddes L A 1991 Handbook of blood pressure measurement. Humana Press, Clifton, NJ

Grap M J 2002 Pulse oximetry. Critical Care Nurse 22(3): 69–76

Gravlee G P, Brockschmidt J K 1990 Accuracy of four indirect methods of blood pressure measurement, with hemodynamic correlations. Journal of Clinical Monitoring 6: 284–298

Hope S A, Tay D B, Meredith I T, Cameron J D 2003 Use of arterial transfer functions for the derivation of aortic waveform characteristics. Journal of Hypertension 21: 1299–1305

Iyriboz Y, Hearon C M, Edwards K 1994 Agreement between large and small cuffs in sphygmomanometry: a quantitative assessment. Journal of Clinical Monitoring 10: 127–133

Kaplan L J, Partland K, Santora T A, Trooskin S Z 2001 Start with a subjective assessment of skin temperatures to identify hypoperfusion in intensive care unit patients. Journal of Trauma 50: 620–628

Korotkoff N S 1905 On the subject of methods of measuring blood pressure. Bulletin of the Imperial Military Medical Academy of St Petersburg

London G E, Blacher J, Pannier B, Guerin A, Marchais S J, Safar M E 2001 Arterial wave reflections and survival in end-stage renal failure. Hypertension 38: 434–438

McAlister F A, Straus S E 2001 Measurement of blood pressure: an evidence based review. British Medical Journal 322: 908–911

McGee D C, Gould M K 2003 Preventing complications of central venous catheterization. New England Journal of Medicine 348: 1123–1133

Mark J B 1995 Getting the most from your central venous pressure catheter. In: Barash P G (ed.) ASA refresher courses in anesthesiology 23. Lippincott-Raven, Philadelphia: 157–175

Mark J B 1998 Atlas of cardiovascular monitoring. Churchill Livingstone, Edinburgh

Mark J B, Slaughter T F, Reves J G 2000 Cardiovascular monitoring. In: Miller R D (ed.) Anesthesia, 5th edn. WB Saunders, Philadelphia: 1117–1206

Merrer J, De Jonghe B, Golliot F et al. 2001 Complication of femoral and subclavian venous catheterization in critically ill patients. JAMA 286: 700–707

Millasseau S C, Patel S J, Redwood S R, Ritter J M, Chowienczyk P J 2003 Pressure wave reflection assessed from the peripheral pulse: is a transfer function necessary? Hypertension 41: 1016–1020

Mitchell G F, Lacourciere Y, Ouellet J P et al. 2003 Determinants of elevated pulse pressure in middle-aged and older subjects with uncomplicated systolic hypertension. Circulation 108: 1592–1598

O'Brien E, Waeber B, Parati G, Staessen J, Myers MG on behalf of the European Society of Hypertension Working Group on Blood Pressure Monitoring 2001 Blood pressure measuring devices: recommendations for the European Society of Hypertension. British Medical Journal 322: 531–536

O'Rourke M F 2003 Arterial pressure waveforms in hypertension. Minerva Medica 94: 229–250

O'Rourke R A, Silverman M E, Schlant R C 1994 General examination of the patient. In: Schlant R C, Alexander R W (eds) The heart: arteries and veins. McGraw-Hill, New York: 238–241

Ostchega Y, Prineas R J, Paulose-Ram R, Grim C M, Willard G, Collins D 2003 The National Health and Nutrition Examination Survey 1999–2000: effect of observer training and protocol standardization on reduction blood pressure error. Journal of Clinical Epidemiology 8: 768–774

Pauca A, O'Rourke M, Kon N 2001 Prospective evaluation of a method for estimating ascending aortic pressure from the radial artery pressure waveform. Hypertension 38: 932–937

Ramsey M 1994 Automatic oscillometric NIBP versus manual auscultatory blood pressure in the PACU. Journal of Clinical Monitoring 10: 136–139

Riva-Rocci S 1887 Un nuovo sfigmomanometro. Gazzetta medica torino 47: 981–996

Seed P 2000 Comparing several methods of measuring the same quantity. Stata Technical Bulletin 55: 2–9

Seeley R R 2000 Anatomy and physiology, 5th edn. WCB McGraw-Hill, California

Sequin P, Rouzo A L, Tanguy M 2000 Evidence for the need of bedside accuracy of pulse oximetry in an intensive care unit. Critical Care Medicine 28: 703–706

Shinozaki T, Deane R S Mazuzan J E 1980 The dynamic responses of liquid-filled catheter systems for direct measurements of blood pressure. Anesthesiology 53: 498–504

Smith G 2000 Acute life threatening event recognition and treatment: a multiprofessional course in care of the acutely ill patient (ALERT). Open Learning, Portsmouth

Smulyan H, Asmar R G, Rudnicki A, London G M, Safar M E 2001 Comparative effect of aging in men and women on the properties of the arterial tree. Journal of the American College of Cardiology 37: 1374–1380

Tensys Medical Inc. 2003 Tensymeter TL-100. Tensys Medical Inc., San Diego, CA

Thaler M S 2003 The only EKG book you'll ever need. Lippincott Williams and Wilkins, Philadelphia

Tisherman S A 2000 Postinjury oxygen consumption: new method, no new answers. Critical Care Medicine 28: 577–578

Van de Louw A, Cracco C, Cerf C et al. 2001 Accuracy of pulse oximetry in the intensive care unit. Intensive Care Medicine 27: 1606–1613

Weber T, Auer J, O'Rourke M F et al 2004 Arterial stiffness, wave reflections and risk of coronary artery disease. Circulation 109: 184–189

White K 2003 Fast facts for adult critical care. Kathy White Learning Systems, Alabama

Wilkinson I B, McCallum H, Flint L, Cockcroft J R, Newby D E, Webb D J 2000 The influence of heart rate on augmentation index and central arterial pressure in humans. Journal of Physiology 525(Part I): 263–270

Young C C, Mark J B, White W et al 1995 Clinical evaluation of continuous non-invasive blood pressure monitoring; accuracy and tracking capabilities. Journal of Clinical Monitoring 11: 245–252

SUGGESTED READING

Benatar S R, Hewlett A M, Nunn J F 1973 The use of iso-shunt lines for control of oxygen therapy. British Journal of Anaesthesia 45: 711–718

Bickler P E, Schapera A, Bainton C R 1990 Acute radial nerve injury from use of an automatic blood pressure monitor. Anesthesiology 3: 186–188

Block F E 1994 What is heart rate anyway? Journal of Clinical Monitoring 10: 366–370

Braunwald E, Fishman A P, Cournand A 1956 Time relationship of dynamic events in the cardiac chambers, pulmonary artery and aorta in man. Circulation Research 4: 100–107

Bruner J M R 1994 On the calibration of artefacts. Journal of Clinical Monitoring 10: 143–146

Case records of the Massachusetts General Hospital 1993 (Case 48) New England Journal of Medicine 329: 1720–1728

Case records of the Massachusetts General Hospital 1996 (Case 1) New England Journal of Medicine 334: 105–111

Cholley B P, Shroff S C, Sandelski J, Erlanger J, Hooker D R 1904 An experimental study of blood pressure and of pulse pressure in man. Johns Hopkins Hospital Report 12: 145–378.

Dauffurn K, Hillman K M, Baumann A, Lum M, Crispin C, Ince L 1994 Fluid balance charts: do they measure up? British Journal of Nursing 3: 816–820

Dautzenberg P L J, Broekman T C J, Hooyer C, Schonwetter R S, Duursma S A 1993 Patient-related predictors of cardiopulmonary resuscitation of hospitalized patients. Age and Ageing 22: 464–475

Franklin C, Mathew J 1994 Developing strategies to prevent in hospital cardiac arrest: Analysing responses of physicians and nurses in the hours before the event. Critical Care Medicine 22: 224–247

Gardner R M 1981 Direct blood pressure measurements – dynamic response requirements. Anesthesiology 54: 227–236

Gardner R M, Hollingsworth K W 1986 Optimizing the electrocardiogram and pressure monitoring. Critical Care Medicine 14: 651–658

Geddes L A 1991 Handbook of blood pressure measurement. Humana Press, Clifton, NJ

Goldhill D R, White S A, Smumner A 1999 Physiological values and procedures in the 24 hours before ICU admission from the ward. Anaesthesia 54: 529–534

Goldhill D R, Worthington L, Mulcahy A, Tarling M, Simner A 1999 The patient at risk team: identifying and managing seriously ill ward patients. Anaesthesia 54: 853–860

Gravlee G P, Brockschmidt J K 1990 Accuracy of four indirect methods of blood pressure measurement, with hemodynamic correlations. Journal of Clinical Monitoring 6: 284–298

Gurushanthaiah K, Weinger M B, Englund C E 1995 Visual display format affects the ability of anesthesiologists to detect acute physiologic changes: a laboratory study employing a clinical display simulator. Anesthesiology 83: 1184–1193

Iyriboz Y, Hearon C M, Edwards K 1994 Agreement between large and small cuffs in sphgmomanometry: a quantitative assessment. Journal of Clinical Monitoring 10: 127–133

Mark J B 1991 The cardiac cycle response. Journal of Cardiothoracic and Vascular Anesthesia 5: 651

O'Rourke M F, Yaginuma T 1984 Wave reflections and the arterial pulse. Archives of International Medicine 144: 366–371

Perloff J K 1987 The clinical recognition of congenital heart disease, 3rd edn. WB Saunders, Philadelphia

Ramsey M 1994 Automatic oscillometric NIBP versus manual auscultatory blood pressure in the PACU. Journal of Clinical Monitoring 10: 136–139

Wallis C B, Davies H T O, Shearer A J 1997 Why do patients die on general wards after discharge from intensive care units? Anaesthesia 52: 9–14

Watson N 1997 Deaths on wards following discharge from the intensive care unit. Anaesthesia 53: 708–709

Weinfurt P T 1990 Electrocardiographic monitoring: an overview. Journal of Clinical Monitoring 6: 132–138

5 Mechanical ventilation

Main objectives

● Outline the effects of mechanical ventilation on the heart and cardiac output, and how these can be used to assess preload.
● Highlight the limitations of pressure measurements to guide therapy in the critically ill by providing an understanding of the relationship between pressure/volume and flow.

Heart–lung interactions

Variations in arterial blood pressure and cardiac output that occur as a result of heart–lung interactions during mechanical ventilation are becoming increasingly valued as clinical observations. This is at a time when minimally invasive methods of measuring cardiac output using pulse contour analysis monitors are being developed (Michard & Teboul 2000, Harrigan & Pinsky 2001a, 2001b, Parry-Jones & Pittman 2003, Teboul 2003). Pulse contour analysis monitors record changes in arterial blood pressure and matches them to the respiratory cycle. The arterial trace is utilized to provide measured variations in systolic pressure, pulse pressure and stroke volume for each respiratory cycle. These variations can then be used in the assessment and management of the hemodynamic status of the patient (Parry-Jones & Pittman 2003, Teboul 2003).

The observation of fluctuations in the arterial blood pressure waveform on a monitor during inspiration and expiration is something that most intensive care nurses are familiar with, and is commonly referred to as a 'respiratory swing'. The magnitude of these fluctuations has always been associated with a patient's state of hydration. Actually, these fluctuations are largely due to alterations in intrathoracic pressure (P_{IT}), which influences the distending pressure of the heart chambers, or transmural pressure (P_{TM}). P_{TM} represents the volume in a chamber (preload) and the resistance it has to pump against (afterload). The P_{TM} is the difference between the pressure measured inside a heart chamber and the P_{IT} outside it. As the P_{IT} rises, the P_{TM} falls (Michard & Teboul 2000, Parry-Jones & Pittman 2003, Teboul 2003)

The respiratory cycle

In order to understand the physiological basis for heart–lung interactions, it is necessary to look at what is happening in the right and left sides of the heart during inspiration and expiration in patients who are on intermittent positive pressure ventilation (IPPV). The mean arterial pressure (MAP) is determined by blood flow and by arterial tone. Arterial pulse pressure, on the other hand, is determined by left ventricular stroke volume, the heart rate and arterial tone. Arterial tone and the heart rate remain fairly constant over the course of a breath. Therefore, arterial pressure variations are mainly due to cyclic changes in stroke volume, caused by the positive pressure breath (Roth-botham et al 1978, Pinsky 1994, Michard & Teboul 2000; Michard et al 2000).

Arterial blood pressure rises on inspiration during IPPV. This rise occurs as a result of several changes taking place. Firstly, the increase in intrathoracic pressure decreases the trans-mural pressure across the left ventricle, whilst at the same time increasing the drainage of blood into the left atrium from the lungs via the pulmonary veins. This increases left ventricular end-diastolic volume (LVEDV) and decreases the tension across the wall of the left ventricle (afterload). As a result, blood is ejected into the systemic circulation more efficiently (Harrigan & Pinsky 2001a, 2001b). At the same time, the increase in intrathoracic pressure reduces venous return (preload) to the right side of the heart (Figures 5.1 and 5.2), reducing the right ventricular end-diastolic volume (RVEDV). In addition, the work of the right ventricle (after-load) is increasing owing to the increase in pulmonary vas-cular resistance (Harrigan & Pinsky 2001a, 2001b).

At the start of expiration, the reduced right ventricular output that occurred during inspiration feeds through to the systemic side of the circulation and the arterial blood pressure starts to fall (the left side of the heart can only eject what is given by the right). Early on in expiration, the increase in transmural pressure reduces pulmonary venous drainage and this results in a further fall in LVEDV (Harri-gan & Pinsky 2001a, 2001b). If full expiration occurs into an apneic period before the next breath, the blood pressure increases again to the baseline value as the improvement in output from the right side of the heart feeds through to the left (Mark 1998, Gunn & Pinsky 2001).

The change in preload that occurs during both inspiration and expiration can affect the performance of the left and

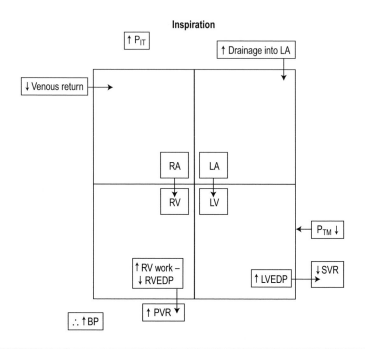

Fig 5.1 Inspiration (see text for details). BP, blood pressure; LA, left atrium; LV, left ventricle; LVEDP, left ventricular end-diastolic pressure; P_{IT}, intrathoracic pressure; P_{TM}, transmural pressure; PVR, peripheral vascular resistance; RA, right atrium; RV, right ventricle; RVEDP, right ventricular end-diastolic pressure; SVR, systemic vascular resistance.

right ventricles during the respiratory cycle because changes in right ventricular preload shifts the septum of the heart over to the left, reducing the compliance of the left ventricle. This results in a reduced LVEDV for the same filling (Michard & Teboul 2000, Harrigan & Pinsky 2001a, 2001b, Parry-Jones & Pittman 2003, Teboul 2003).

Systolic pressure variation, pulse pressure variation and stroke volume variation

Systolic pressure variation (SPV) is calculated across a respiratory cycle from the minimum and maximum systolic

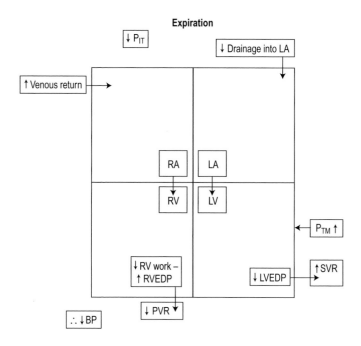

Fig 5.2 Expiration (see text for details). BP, blood pressure; LA, left atrium; LV, left ventricle; LVEDP, left ventricular end-diastolic pressure; P_{IT}, intrathoracic pressure; P_{TM}, transmural pressure; PVR, peripheral vascular resistance; RA, right atrium; RV, right ventricle; RVEDP, right ventricular end-diastolic pressure; SVR, systemic vascular resistance.

pressure at end expiration. Pulse pressure is the systolic pressure minus the diastolic blood pressure. Pulse pressure variation (PPV) is the variation in this measurement over the respiratory cycle (Beaussier et al 1995, Rook et al 1995, Tavernier 1998). Preload and afterload change during the respiratory cycle, and alterations in left ventricular output (stroke volume) occur. Stroke volume variation (SVV) is determined by the magnitude of these changes (Gunn & Pinsky 2001).

During a period of apnea, a baseline measurement of systolic pressure is taken. This provides the reference point when looking at the increase in systolic pressure during inspiration and the decrease in systolic pressure during expiration. The degree of variation between the two reflects the proportion of increase and decrease in right and left ventricular preload, and the reduction in left ventricular afterload. This may indicate a patient's ability to respond to a fluid challenge (Gunn & Pinsky 2001, Parry-Jones & Pittman 2003, Teboul 2003, Wiesenack et al 2003). The minimum and maximum intrathoracic pressure during a respiratory cycle is not known and has a variable effect on SPV. It is possible that this variation is, in fact, due to transmitted airway pressure rather than preload. PPV; however, it is measured at the same intrathoracic pressure, so it is not affected by these changes. For this reason, PPV may be more reliable as a preload indicator (Parry-Jones & Pittman 2003, Teboul 2003, Wiesenack et al 2003).

As preload and afterload change throughout the respiratory cycle, output from the left ventricle will move up and down the Starling curve. A total systolic pressure variation of 10 mmHg (5 cm up and 5 cm down from the baseline) is seen normally in mechanically ventilated patients. However, a change in systolic pressure greater than 5 cm H_2O down from the baseline measurement indicates hypovolemia and is a good predictor of preload dependence. However, a pulse pressure variation greater than 13% may be more reliable (Harrigan & Pinsky 2001a, 2001b).

For the reliable measurement of SPV, PPV and, in particular, SVV, it is recommended that patients be ventilated with a tidal volume and respiratory rate that is constant. There are two reasons for this. Firstly, self-ventilating patients have considerable variability in respiratory rates and tidal volumes, making it difficult to obtain an accurate measure. Secondly, the changes seen in arterial pressure throughout the respiratory cycle are opposite to those seen in patients on IPPV. As yet, it is not clear from the literature if SPV or

PPV can be used in these situations (Parry-Jones & Pittman 2003). SPV and PPV may be affected by changes in PEEP, chest or lung compliance, large tidal volumes or high respiratory rates by intermittently increasing intrathoracic pressure. Importantly, on a beat-by-beat basis, it is the changes in left ventricular stroke volume that cause a variation in arterial pulse pressure. Having said that, over time, other factors can affect it, such as vascular tone and arterial resistance/elastance (Michard & Teboul 2000, Parry-Jones & Pittman 2003, Marx et al 2004).

Pulse pressure variation

Positive pressure ventilation transiently increases the pressure in the thorax (intrathoracic pressure), altering stroke volume and decreasing preload. This can be seen reflected on the arterial pressure waveform as a variation in pressure, which mirrors the respiratory cycle (Jardin et al 1983, Gunn & Pinsky 2001). The ability to measure this arterial pressure variation (either pulse pressure or systolic pressure) allows the prediction of not only the patients' cardiovascular response, but also the degree of response to changes in their intravascular volume (we will return to this in Chapter 6). Mean arterial pressure is determined by blood flow and by arterial tone. Arterial pulse pressure is determined by left ventricular stroke volume, heart rate and arterial tone (Pinsky et al 1991, Pinsky 1994). Over the course of a breath, the heart rate and arterial tone remain fairly constant; therefore, variations in arterial pressure are mainly due to transient changes in stroke volume, induced by the positive pressure breath (Pinsky 2003b, Fawcett 2004). Importantly, on a beat-to-beat basis, it is only changes in left ventricular stroke volume that cause a variation in arterial pulse pressure (over time factors such as vascular tone, arterial resistance/elastance can influence it) (Figure 5.3).

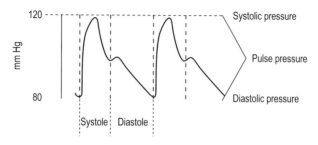

Fig 5.3 Pulse pressure variation. (Reproduced with permission from Mark 1998.)

Systolic pressure variation

Systolic pressure variation is the variation in the systolic pressure reading following a positive pressure breath. It is the difference between the maximum and minimum systolic pressure recorded over the respiratory cycle (Perel & Pizov 1992, Beaussier et al 1995, Gunn & Pinsky 2001). Although the actual mechanism behind the initial increase in systolic pressure is unproven, the likely cause is thought to be as a result of alterations in transpulmonary pressure that are associated with positive pressure breathing (causing a slight increase in left ventricular preload) and as a consequence of increased intrathoracic pressure (decreasing left ventricular afterload). The total systolic pressure variation can be divided into an increase in pressure that occurs early in inspiration, referred to as the delta up, and a decrease in pressure that occurs later, referred to as the delta down (Parry-Jones & Pittman 2003). The delta up reflects the increase in left ventricular output during inspiration and the delta down reflects the degree of systemic venous return impairment that becomes evident in the arterial pressure trace shortly afterwards. A total systolic pressure variation of 10 mmHg (5 mmHg delta up and 5 mmHg delta down) is seen normally in mechanically ventilated patients (Figure 5.4; Parry-Jones & Pittman 2003).

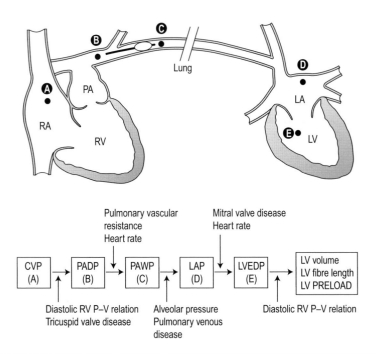

Fig 5.4 Pressure measurements as surrogates for left ventricular preload. CVP, central venous pressure; LAP, left atrial pressure; LA, left atrium; LV, left ventricle; LVEDP, left ventricular end-diastolic pressure; PA, pulmonary artery; PADP, pulmonary artery diastolic pressure; PAWP, pulmonary artery wedge pressure; RA, right atrium; RV, right ventricle. (Reproduced with permission from Mark 1998.)

The shape of the arterial pressure waveform is mainly affected by the deflection of pressure waves as blood travels from the aorta into the peripheral circulation. The mean arterial pressure falls only slightly as blood flows from the aorta to, say, the radial artery. This is because there is only a modest amount of resistance to blood flow (Mark 1998, Pauca et al, 2001). Once the flow of blood reaches the arterioles, the mean arterial pressure falls significantly because of a marked increase in resistance in these vessels. Having said that, although the increased resistance to flow causes a decrease in pulsatile pressure downstream, it causes the pressure pulsations upstream to increase because of the

> ## Quiz 5.1
>
> 1. What is the effect on cardiac output during systole in the mechanically ventilated patient? Why does this occur?
>
> 2. Do you know what systolic pulse and stroke variations are? What causes them and how are they clinically relevant?

deflection of the pressure wave (Harrigan & Pinsky 2001a,b).

Stroke volume variation

The stroke volume variation is the mean difference (as measured) between the highest and lowest stroke volume over the last 30 s. The stroke volume changes with respiration in the same way as pulse and systolic pressures. It rises on inspiration with venous return and falls on expiration, against venous return. Positive pressure ventilation affects venous return by reducing it; therefore, in mechanically ventilated patients, the stroke volume variation is likely to be greater in patients who are dehydrated. This is because the heart is unable to compensate for the changes in stroke volume throughout the respiratory cycle (inspiration and expiration), if there is insufficient blood volume to compensate for it (Michard & Teboul 2000, 2002).

The evidence

Evidence exists suggesting the use of heart–lung interactions as a tool in cardiovascular monitoring broadly in two situations. Firstly, to find out if flow (cardiac output) has been improved as a result of a fluid challenge and, secondly, as a means of predicting whether increasing preload will, in fact, improve cardiac output (Harrigan & Pinsky 2001a,b). However, it should be remembered that patients should be ventilated with a tidal volume of 10 ml/kg for these heart–lung interactions to be useful clinically. To date, SPV has been used most frequently clinically, firstly, as a means of identifying when a patient is hypovolemic. It has been used, secondly, for monitoring the subsequent volume resuscitation, where SPV has been found to be more effective in the identification or prediction of hypovolemia than mean arterial blood pressure, central venous pressure, pulmonary artery occlusion pressure or left ventricular end-diastolic area index. This has been found to be true even when arterial blood pressure is maintained at near-normal levels and when referenced against echocardiography (Michard & Teboul, 2000, Harrigan & Pinsky 2001a, 2001b, Parry-Jones & Pittman 2003, Teboul 2003). In sepsis-related hypotension, the SPV has showed a significant response to fluid challenges.

However, despite the evidence, the use of SPV, PPV or SVV for monitoring and detecting hypovolemia in a wide variety of settings has yet to be proven, in particular, for patients with low and variable tidal volumes (Feissel et al 2000, Parry-Jones & Pittman 2003).

Intermittent positive pressure ventilation brings about cyclic changes in left ventricular stroke volume (highest during inspiration, lowest during expiration). These changes relate mainly to the decrease on expiration in left ventricular preload owing to the decrease on inspiration in ejection from the right ventricle (Michard et al 2000).

The prediction of left ventricular end-diastolic pressure

The whole point of pulmonary artery pressure monitoring is to measure hemodynamic parameters that can be used to estimate left ventricular filling pressures, which will then help to guide the administration of fluids and vasoactive drugs, particularly when clinical signs, symptoms and other monitored variables are not useful clinically. The reason for wanting an accurate estimate of left ventricular end-diastolic pressure is that we want to know if the patient is developing pulmonary edema (Calvin et al 1981, Gunn & Pinsky 2001). The filling pressure actually provides an estimate of the hydrostatic pressure in the pulmonary capillaries that represents the vascular back pressure consistent with the formation of pulmonary edema. This is reflected in the pulmonary artery wedge pressure. The wedge pressure and the capillary pressure are not the same thing (Mark 1998, Fawcett 2004).

Generally, the pulmonary capillary wedge pressure (PCWP) is reported as a mean pressure; an end-diastolic component of wedge pressure can be identified as well as its phasic pressure trace. In normal sinus rhythm, atrial contraction provides this mechanical end-diastolic event. Therefore, the measurement of the pulmonary capillary wedge pressure a-wave pressure peak gives a more accurate estimation of left ventricular end-diastolic pressure than that of the mean pulmonary capillary wedge pressure. The mean wedge pressure is not always equal to the end-diastolic pressure value and, the taller the a- and v-waves, the greater may be the discrepancy. This is important (Mark 1998).

Underestimation or overestimation of left ventricular end-diastolic pressure is common in certain conditions (Tables 5.1 and 5.2). The problem is greater if patients have multiple pathologies.

Table 5.1 Underestimation of left ventricular end-diastolic pressure. (Reproduced with permission from Mark 1998)

Condition	Discrepancy	Cause
Decreased left ventricular compliance	Mean LAP < LVEDP	Increased end-diastolic a-wave
Aortic valve regurgitation	LAP a-wave < LVEDP	Mitral wave closure prior to end-diastole
Pulmonary valve regurgitation	PADP < LVEDP	Bidirectional runoff for pulmonary artery flow
Right bundle branch block	PADP < LVEDP	Delayed pulmonary valve opening
Decreased pulmonary vascular bed	PAWP < LVEDP	Obstruction of pulmonary blood flow

LAP, left atrial pressure; LVEDP, left ventricular end-diastolic pressure; PADP, pulmonary artery diastolic pressure; PAWP, pulmonary artery wedge pressure.

The relationship between pressure and volume

The aim of monitoring central circulatory pressures it to give us some idea of the volume status of patients, which enables us to ensure critically ill patients have adequate circulatory volumes. Ideally, the volume of the ventricles would be monitored continuously in critically ill patients. However, this has not been the case historically (the alternative methods of estimating ventricular volumes will be discussed in Chapter 6).

Targeting and measuring hemodynamic end-points

As indicators of patient's cardiovascular status, intravascular filling pressures have repeatedly been shown to be

Table 5.2 Overestimation of left ventricular end-diastolic pressure. (Reproduced with permission from Mark 1998)

Condition	Discrepancy	Cause
Positive end-expiratory pressure	Mean PAWP > mean LAP	Creation of lung zone 1 or 2 pericardial pressure changes
Pulmonary arterial hypertension	PADP > mean PAWP	Increased pulmonary vascular resistance
Pulmonary veno-occlusive disease	Mean PAWP > mean LAP	Obstruction to flow in large pulmonary veins
Mitral valve stenosis	Mean LAP > LVEDP	Obstruction to flow across mitral valve
Mitral valve regurgitation	Mean LAP > LVEDP	Systolic v-wave raises mean arterial pressure
Tachycardia	PADP > mean LAP > LVEDP	Short diastole creates pulmonary vascular and mitral valve gradients
Ventricular septal defect	Mean LAP > LVEDP	Systolic v-wave raises mean arterial pressure

LAP, left atrial pressure; LVEDP, left ventricular end-diastolic pressure; PADP, pulmonary artery diastolic pressure; PAWP, pulmonary artery wedge pressure.

unreliable (Parry-Jones & Pittman 2003), and data are available to demonstrate that changes in pressure and changes in flow have a poor correlation (Teboul 2003). However, pressure measurements, such as arterial blood pressure (ABP), central venous pressure (CVP) and PCWP, are still being relied upon as indicators of hydration and perfusion. Physiologically the body's compensatory mechanisms preserve pressure at the expense of flow; therefore, they maintain arterial blood pressure despite cardiovascular fluid volume depletion. Thus, the use of bedside indicators of right ventricular (CVP) and left ventricular (PCWP) preload are still used to guide fluid therapy because many patients with circulatory failure do respond positively to fluid therapy despite a lack of indication of hypovolemia clinically (Kincaid et al 2001, Michard & Teboul 2002, Leeper 2003).

The ventricles of most healthy individuals function on the ascending portion of the Starling curve, so that any changes in intravascular volume will increase stroke volume. Such individuals are said to be responders or preload dependent. However, 50% of patients in circulatory failure have ventricles that operate on the flat portion of the Starling curve. For these patients, an increase in intravascular volume may be detrimental, and they are said to be non-responders or preload independent. The difficulty lies in identifying who falls into which category. In order to manage a patient's hemodynamic status safely, we need to know which patients are already filled, so that fluid is not given inappropriately. We need to know if patients need inotropes and what is happening in the systemic circulation (e.g. do they need vasoconstricting or vasodilating?). For these reasons, it is important to identify the factors that will accurately predict who does and who does not require fluid (Michard & Teboul 2000, Teboul 2003).

The PCWP is used most often in the assessment of pulmonary edema, pulmonary vasomotor tone, intravascular volume status, left ventricular preload and left ventricular performance (Pinsky 2003a). Its ability to accurately assess intravascular volume is in question. This is because it is subject to the most error in its measurement and interpretation and, for multiple reasons related to determinants of left ventricular compliance and resistance, it is the least accurate (Brock, 2002, Pinsky 2003).

The pulmonary artery catheter estimates the preload of both the right and left ventricles by relying on the hemodynamic monitoring of cardiac filling pressures. This estimate of left ventricular end-diastolic pressure (LVEDP) or pulmonary artery wedge pressure is based on the assumption that changes in filling pressure directly reflect changes (in proportion and in the same direction) in filling volume. However, because the relationship between pressure and volume is not linear (characterized by a straight line), but curvilinear (characterized by a curved line), this is not the case. In fact, diastolic pressure and volume can alter in opposite directions to each other (Mark 1998). Therefore, it cannot be assumed that a proportional change in ventricular preload has occurred just because there has been a change in the central venous or pulmonary artery wedge pressure measurement obtained.

The relationship between filling pressure and filling volume depends on which portion of the ventricular diastolic pressure–volume curve at which the patient's ventricle is operating (Starling 1896). For example, a significant increase in preload (filling volume) can be associated with only a moderate increase in filling pressures when the ventricle is operating on the flat portion of the curve. However, if the ventricle is operating on the sharp portion of the curve, there is little influence on preload for the same increase in the filling pressures measured (Figure 5.5). In the case of cardiac compromise, for example, the onset of cardiac ischemia, the relationship between the end-diastolic ventricular pressure and end-diastolic volume changes. This can result in an increase in the end-diastolic filling pressure measured with an associated reduction in filling volume or vice versa. This makes accurate assessment of the patient's left ventricular end-diastolic volume even more difficult (Mark 1998, Kincaid et al 2001, Parry-Jones & Pittman 2003).

Pressure and volume loops are simply graphical representations of the function of both the right and left ventricles,

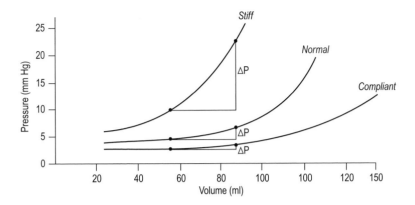

Fig 5.5 The shape of the ventricular diastolic pressure–volume curve determines the relationship between a given change in measured pressure and the corresponding change in ventricular volume. In this example, for the same change in ventricular volume from 55 to 85 ml, the change measured in measured filling pressure (ΔP) will be 12, 2 or 1 mmHg, depending on whether the ventricle is 'stiff', 'normal' or 'compliant', respectively.

showing how the relationship between pressure and volume can change in different circumstances, depending on the cardiac properties of an individual patient (Mark 1998). A change in the relationship between pressure and volume, as reflected in a diastolic pressure and volume curve, occurs as a result of a number of factors. For example, changes in the internal properties of the ventricle, such as its compliance (otherwise known as the stiffness, ability to distend or its elastance), its shape and its ability to relax. External factors can also influence the pressure–volume relationship (e.g. the pericardium, the pleural pressure, the right ventricle and the coronary circulation). It is important to take these factors into account when looking at the relationship between pressure and volume to avoid making misleading judgments (Buda et al 1979, Michard et al 2000).

Measuring left ventricular preload using central venous pressure

It makes sense that the further away from the left ventricular end-diastolic pressure site, the less likely a precise measurement or estimate can be made. Reliance on the central venous pressure as an estimate of left ventricular preload can be misleading in critically ill patients. This is because two factors can affect its accuracy: the interdependence and the constraint exerted by the pericardium (Pinsky 2003b). These make the central venous pressure problematic as a surrogate for left ventricular preload for several reasons (Mark 1998). Firstly, the left and right ventricles are joined together by the septum. Secondly, both ventricles are also restricted by the pericardium that surrounds them. This makes the left and right ventricles dependent on each other (Parry-Jones & Pitman 2003). As a result, the pressure and volume relation occurring in the left ventricle is affected by what is happening in the right, creating additional interpretive problems. A good example of this is when an increase in the end-diastolic pressure occurs in the left ventricle, with a lower increase in volume, as a direct result of the interventricular septum shifting over to the left (Mark 1998). This occurs in acute pulmonary hypertension, when right ventricular end-diastolic pressure and volume increase (Pagel et al 1993a, 1993b, Pinsky 2003b).

Measurement of the transmural pressure would be the ideal. However, it is difficult to measure easily or accurately, which is why reliance is put on intravascular pressure measurements as a substitute. Ventricular preload, end-diastolic volumes and the length of the myocardial fibers influence the pressures recorded inside the heart because the chambers are within the thorax and surrounded by the pericardium. Obviously, any change in the structures that surround the heart will affect the accuracy of any readings recorded (Mark 1998, Pinsky 2003b).

Measuring left ventricular preload using the pulmonary artery wedge pressure

Ordinarily, the value accepted or aimed for in a pressure measurement is based on our knowledge of the patient's pre-existing disease state, and an assumption being made about the pericardial pressure and stiffness of the heart chambers during diastole. This is particularly true when the pulmonary artery wedge pressure is being utilized as a measure of preload. There is a delicate balance between adequate preload and the prevention of the development of hydrostatic pulmonary edema. Obviously, a lower wedge pressure value would be aimed for in patients who have existing pulmonary damage than in patients with existing myocardial damage (Mark 1998).

When the wedge pressure is high or low, it makes sense to alter the value to avoid pulmonary edema while improving cardiac output. Critically ill patients pose real problems in this area and predicting an optimum value is difficult, often requiring a trial fluid bolus (the amount depends on the patient's pre-existing pathology) of crystalloid over a short period of time (15 min or so) and assessing the patient's response (Pinsky 2003a).

REFERENCES

Beaussier M, Coriat P, Perel A et al 1995 Determinants of systolic pressure variation in patients ventilated after vascular surgery. Journal of Cardiothoracic and Vascular Anesthesia 9: 547–551

Brock H, Gabriel C, Bibl D, Necek D 2002 Monitoring intravascular volumes for postoperative volume therapy. European Journal of Anaesthesiology 19: 288–294

Buda A J, Pinsky M R, Ingels N B et al 1979 Effect of intrathoracic pressure on the left ventricular performance. New England Journal of Medicine 301: 453–459

Calvin J E, Driedger A A, Sibbald W J 1981 Does the pulmonary capillary wedge pressure predict left ventricular preload in critically ill patients? Critical Care Medicine 9: 437–443

Fawcett J A D 2004 Haemodynamic monitoring: heart–lung interactions. Care of the Critically Ill 20(2): 38–41

Feissel M, Michard F, Mangin I, Ruyer O, Faller J P, Teboul J L 2001 Respiratory changes in aortic blood velocity as an indicator of fluid responsiveness in ventilated patients with septic shock. Chest 119: 867–873

Gunn S R, Pinsky M R 2001 Implications of arterial pressure variation in patients in the intensive care unit. Current Opinion in Critical Care 7: 212–217

Harrigan P, Pinsky M 2001a Heart–lung interactions. Part 1: effects of lung volumes and ventilation. International Journal of Intensive Care 8: 6–13

Harrigan P, Pinsky M 2001b Heart–lung interactions. Part 2: effects of intra-thoracic pressure. International Journal of Intensive Care 8: 99–108

Jardin F, Farcot J C, Gueret P et al 1983 Cyclic changes in arterial pulse during respiratory support. Circulation 68: 266–274

Kincaid E H, Meredith W, Chang M C 2001 Determining optimal cardiac preload during resuscitation using measurement of ventricular compliance. Journal of Trauma 50: 665–669

Leeper B 2003 Monitoring right ventricular volumes: a paradigm shift. AACN Clinical Issues 14: 208–219.

Mark J B 1998 Atlas of cardiovascular monitoring. Churchill Livingstone, Edinburgh

Marx G, Cope T, McCrossan L et al 2004 Assessing fluid responsiveness by stroke volume variation in mechanically ventilated patients with severe sepsis. European Journal of Anaesthesiology 21: 132–138

Michard F, Boussat S, Chemla D et al 2000 Relation between respiratory changes in arterial pulse pressure and fluid responsiveness in septic patients with acute circulatory failure. American Journal of Respiratory and Critical Care Medicine 162: 134–138

Michard F, Teboul J L 2000 Using heart–lung interactions to assess fluid responsiveness during mechanical ventilation. Critical Care 4: 282–289

Michard F, Teboul J L 2002 Predicting fluid responsiveness in ICU patients. Chest 121: 2000–2008

Pagel P S, Grossman W, Haering J M, Warltier D S 1993a Left ventricular diastolic function in the normal and diseased heart. Perspectives for the anesthesioligst. [First of two parts.] Anesthesiology 79: 836–854

Pagel P S, Grossman W, Haering J M, Warltier D C 1993b Left ventricular diastolic function in the normal and diseased heart. Perspectives for the anaesthesiologist. [Second of two parts.] Anesthesiology 79: 1104–1120

Parry-Jones A J D, Pittman J A L 2003 Arterial pressure and stroke volume variability as measurements for cardiovascular optimisation. International Journal of Intensive Care 10: 2

Pauca A, O'Rourke M, Kon N 2001 Prospective evaluation of a method for estimating ascending aortic pressure from the radial artery pressure waveform. Hypertension 38: 932–937

Perel A, Pizov R 1992 Cardiovascular effects of mechanical ventilation. In: Perel A, Stock M C (eds) Handbook of mechanical ventilatory support. Williams & Wilkins, Baltimore: 51–65

Pinsky M R 1994 Cardiovascular effects of ventilatory support and withdrawal. Anesthesia Analogues 79: 567–576

Pinsky M R 2003a Pulmonary artery wedge pressure. Intensive Care Medicine 29:19–22

Pinsky M R 2003b Clinical significance of pulmonary artery occlusion pressure. Intensive Care Medicine 29: 175–178

Pinsky M, Vincent J L, De Smet J M 1991 Estimating left ventricular filling pressure during positive end-expiratory pressure in humans. American Review of Respiratory Disease 143: 25–31

Robotham J L, Lixfeld W, Holland L et al 1978 Effects of respiration on cardiac performance. Journal of Applied Physiology 44: 703–709

Rook G A, Schwid H A, Shapira Y 1995 The effect of graded haemorrhage and intravascular volume replacement on systolic pressure variation in humans during mechanical and spontaneous ventilation. Anesthesia Analogues 80: 925–932

Starling E H 1896 On the absorption of fluids from the connective tissue spaces. Journal of Physiology 9: 312

Tavernier B, Makhotine O, Lebuffe G 1998 Systolic pressure variation as a guide to fluid therapy in patients with sepsis-induced hypotension. Anaesthesiology 89: 1313–1321

Teboul J L 2003 Dynamic concepts of volume responsiveness. International Journal of Intensive Care 10: 2

Wiesenack C, Prasser C, Rodig G, Kely C 2003 Stroke volume variation as an indicator of fluid responsiveness using pulse contour analysis in mechanically ventilated patients. Cardiovascular Anaesthesia 96: 1254–1257

SUGGESTED READING

Bergquist B D, Bellows W H, Leung J M 1996 Transesophageal echocardiography in myocardial revascularization. II Influence on intraoperative decision making. Anesthesia Analogues 82: 1139–1145

Berkenstadt H, Margalit N, Hadani M, Friedman Z, Segal E, Perel A 2001 Stroke volume variation as a predictor of fluid responsiveness in patients undergoing brain surgery. Anesthesia Analogues 92: 984–989

Case records of the Massachusetts General Hospital (Case 48 1993) New England Journal of Medicine 329: 1720–1728

Case records of the Massachusetts General Hospital (Case 1 1996). New England Journal of Medicine 334: 105–111

Cozzi P J, Hall J B, Schmidt G A 1995 Pulmonary artery diastolic-occlusion pressure gradient is increased in acute pulmonary embolism. Critical Care Medicine 23: 1481–1484

Jardin F, Farcot J C, Gueret P et al 1983 Cyclic changes in arterial pulse during respiratory support. Circulation 68: 266–274

Kushwaha S S, Fallon J T, Fuster V 1997 Restrictive cardiomyopathy. New England Journal of Medicine 336: 267–276

Robotham J L, Cherry D, Mitzner W et al 1983 A re-evaluation of the hemodynamic consequences of intermittent positive pressure ventilation. Critical Care Medicine 11: 783–793

Robotham J L, Scharf S M 1983 Effects of positive and negative pressure ventilation on cardiac performance. Clinical Chest Medicine 4: 161–187

Roizen M F, Berger D L, Gabel R A et al 1993 Practice guidelines for pulmonary artery catheterisation. A report by the American Society of Anesthesiologists task force on pulmonary artery catheterisation. Anesthesiology 78: 380–394

Clinical scenario 2

George Ingleton is a 55-year-old gentleman who has no signifi-cant previous medical history. He was admitted to the critical care unit yesterday with sepsis following an untreated urinary tract infection. He is ventilated on pressure-controlled ventilation ($25\,cmH_2O$) with a positive end-expiratory pressure (PEEP) of $8\,cmH_2O$. He is sedated but very agitated on the ventilator.

You have just taken over his care on the night shift. You were told at handover that he had been hypotensive (95/60) for much of the afternoon despite a total of 1500 ml in fluid (colloid and crystalloid). He has an arterial line and a central venous pressure (CVP) line. However, the traces are not very good.

- Have this gentleman's homeostatic mechanisms been triggered?
- How do you know?
- How would you assess the accuracy of all the monitoring systems in use in this scenario?
- How might you optimize the data generated by the monitoring systems in use?
- What further information would help you to assess his central and peripheral perfusion?

For answers, see Appendix 2 (page 233).

Making the most of hemodynamic technologies to treat the critically ill

Technology

Main objectives

- Describe the history behind technology development.
- Describe how cardiac output can be estimated clinically.
- Differentiate between the types of technology available to measure and monitor central pressures/volumes and flow.
- Provide an understanding of the theories that underpin each of the technologies described.
- Outline the principles underpinning a range of hemodynamic monitors.
- Identify the parameters each technology measures.
- List the advantages and disadvantages of each monitoring system.
- Identify the potential uses of each monitor in different clinical situations.

Technologies for measuring cardiac output

The specific aims of monitoring are that they are initiated at the earliest possible time in order to provide prompt recognition of circulatory problems, from admission to the critical care unit or, preferably, the onset of critical illness (Pittman & Gupta 2003).

Since Swan, Ganz and colleagues introduced the balloon-tipped thermodilution pulmonary artery catheter in the 1970s (Swan et al 1970), it has been used for circulatory measurements and has remained the gold standard for the evaluation of circulatory dysfunction. Initially, use of the catheter was focused on the measurement of pulmonary artery and pulmonary artery wedge pressures, with the estimation of cardiac output being a later development. The pulmonary artery catheter continues to be used in clinical practice (Afessa et al 2001; Pittman & Gupta 2003). However, this method of evaluating circulatory dysfunction is both time consuming and labor intensive (medical and nursing), and not without risks to the patient (Stetz et al 1982, Kadota 1986, Connors et al 1996, Dalen & Bone 1996, Bernard et al 2000).

The ideal method of cardiac output monitoring should produce a continuous display of information that is useful clinically, as well as being non-invasive, reproducible, inexpensive, user friendly, in reasonable agreement with thermodilution results and acceptable to patients (Fawcett 2003). As with all monitoring and imaging techniques, motion, anxiety, restlessness, shivering, agitation and hyperventilation can not only interfere with the measurements obtained, but can also increase the patient's own physiologic responses. A 15% difference between invasive and non-invasive cardiac output estimations are considered acceptable when substantial changes from the normal range are present. Thermodilution also has inaccuracies in both high and low cardiac output ranges, often as a result of operator error or errors from injectate temperature calibration. This is especially true when the patient has hypothermia and is shivering, anxious or has dysrhythmias (Tuman et al 1989b, Sandham et al 2003).

Technology and techniques that provide additional parameters that are not obtainable from the pulmonary artery catheter have been developed, as well as less invasive techniques in cardiac output estimation (Figure 6.1). These are generating increasing interest from intensivists the world over and are becoming much more widely used in practice as alternatives (Pittman & Gupta 2003).

Several technologies and techniques are available (Pittman & Gupta 2003). Generally, they take less time and resources to establish than the pulmonary artery catheter (most, but not all, can be set up and managed by nurses alone) and, more importantly, represent less risk to patients who are already compromised by their critical illness (Fawcett 2003, McKendry et al 2004). Most are still invasive to varying degrees, although some more so than others, requiring

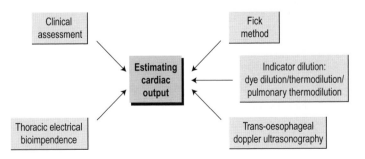

Fig 6.1 A logical grouping of the theories underpinning the technologies that measure cardiac output.

sedation and/or mechanical ventilation, and either arterial and/or central venous access (Tables 6.1 and 6.2). Many of the patients in intensive care will have at least one of these (Headley 1998, Ott et al 2001).

These techniques do not exclude each other because their advantages and limitations are quite different. They are also not intended to replace the pulmonary artery catheter, which continues to be unique in providing pressures (right atrial, pulmonary artery and pulmonary 'wedged' pressures) as well as venous oxygen saturation, in addition to cardiac output. These parameters are still thought of as useful in the management of critically ill patients. These emerging technologies and techniques will now be considered in detail.

Table 6.1 Characteristics of hemodynamic monitors

Monitor	Invasiveness time to set-up	Workload involved	Beat to beat	Inaccuracies
LiDCO	++ Any arterial catheter and site	++ Lithium dilution calibration	Yes	Significant SVR changes
PiCCO	+++ Femoral or brachial arterial line	++ Thermodilution calibration	Yes	Significant SVR changes
CardiacQ	++ Esophageal probe	+++ Probe adjustment	Yes	Fluid loading, increased CO
NICO	+ Non-invasive	++ Rebreathing periods	No	Rapid changes in CVS, low TVs
BioZ	+ Non-invasive	Minimal	Yes	High levels of lung water

CO, cardiac output; CVS, cardiovascular system; SVR, systemic vascular resistance; TV, tidal volume.

Table 6.2 Additional hemodynamic parameters				
Monitor	**Preload**	**Afterload**	**Contractility**	**Other**
LiDCO	SVV, SPV, PPV			
PiCCO	SVV, SPV, GEDV, ITBV	SVR	GEF, CFI	EVLW, PVPI
CardiacQ	FTc, LVETc	SVR, TSVR	PV, MA	AD, ABF
NICO		SVR		PCBF, Vd/Vt
BioZ	LVET	SVR	VI, AI	TFC

ABF, descending aortic blood flow; AD, aortic diameter; AI, acceleration index; CFI, cardiac function index; EVLW, extravascular lung water; FTc, flow time; GEDV, global end-diastolic volume; GEF, global ejection fraction; ITBV, intrathoracic blood volume; LVET, left ventricular ejection time; LVETc, corrected left ventricular ejection time; MA, mean acceleration; PCBF, pulmonary capillary blood flow; PPV, pulse pressure variation; PV, PVPI, pulmonary vascular permeability index; SPV, systolic pressure variation; SVR, systemic vascular resistance; SVV, stroke volume variation; TFC, thoracic fluid content; TSVR, total systemic vascular resistance; Vd/Vt, ratio of physiological dead space to tidal volume; VI, velocity index.

Cardiac output assessed 'clinically'

This method of cardiac output estimation is by the clinical assessment of patients by nursing or medical staff using a two-stage process. This method was proposed and has been evaluated by the medical and nursing team on the intensive care unit at Guy's and St Thomas' Hospital in London, England (Treacher et al 1994, Thomson et al 1996, Creed 2000).

Firstly, the estimation of systemic vascular resistance is made using an initial assessment of temperature change in specific sites on the patient (e.g. toe, ankle, knee, thigh, finger, wrist, elbow and upper arm on each side of the body). Each site is assigned numeric 'Wood' units, which are then converted to dynes/s per cm^5 by multiplying by

79.9. All limbs are assessed to take into account the environment and clinical factors. Depending on the degree of temperature change at each site, from warm to cold, a Wood unit value is assigned to it (the lower the Wood unit, the more normal the systemic vascular resistance is deemed to be).

Secondly, stroke volume is clinically estimated by taking the 'best central pulse' (carotid, brachial or femoral) felt on the patient. For example, if the central pulse cannot be palpated or is hard to establish, the stroke volume is estimated to be 0–20 ml. If it is weak but can be detected, the stroke volume is estimated to be 30–50 ml. A 'normal' pulse that is neither weak or bounding is estimated to be 60–70 ml, whereas a full and bounding central pulse would estimate the stroke volume to be 80–100 ml.

If both the two stages corroborate with each other, the estimates are then accepted and cardiac output can be calculated by multiplying the estimated stroke volume by the patient's heart rate (Creed 2000).

The equation used for this method of estimating non-invasive cardiac output is based on three main factors that influence it. Two of these factors are stroke volume and heart rate. The third factor is related to cardiac output distribution or 'flow'. This flow is said to be determined by mean arterial pressure (MAP) or driving pressure, central venous pressure (CVP) or resisting pressure, and resistance to flow, the systemic vascular resistance (SVR). The equation is:

$$\text{Flow rate} = \frac{\text{Mean arterial pressure} - \text{mean venous pressure}}{\text{Systemic vascular resistance}}$$

Therefore, the estimate depends on the accurate assessment of either the systemic vascular resistance and/or the flow rate (cardiac output). The emphasis of this method is on its ability to determine whether the patient's cardiac output is high, low or normal, using simple non-invasive clinical assessment (Treacher et al 1994, Thomson et al 1996, Creed 2000).

Pulmonary artery catheterization

The pulmonary artery catheter directly measures the pulmonary artery and pulmonary artery wedge pressures, to assess left ventricular filling pressure. In the normal heart, left ventricular pressure is within approximately 2 mmHg of the pulmonary artery wedge pressure, which, in turn, approximates the left ventricular end-diastolic pressure (Mark 1998, Leatherman & Shapiro 2003, Pinsky 2003a).

Floating the pulmonary artery catheter

The process of preparing for and inserting the catheter, obtaining pulmonary artery pressure and successfully wedging the device, can be time consuming and labor intensive. It is important that all the equipment needed is set up correctly, and that the potential problems as well as their solutions are known prior to the start of the procedure, to keep delays to a minimum. This is particularly true if the patient is awake and aware of what is going on (Fawcett 2003).

Prior to pulmonary artery catheter flotation, proper assembly and functioning of the catheter and pressure monitoring system must be confirmed (Figure 6.2). Each lumen should be flushed (usually with saline) and the balloon checked to make sure that it will inflate, ensuring that the balloon surrounding the tip of the catheter is not obstructing the distal lumen. The assembly of the catheter-monitoring system can be achieved using a simple method.

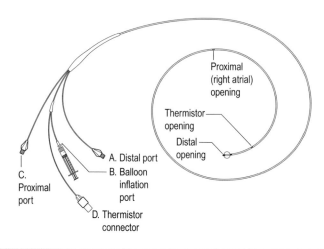

Fig 6.2 Quadruple-lumen thermodilution pulmonary artery catheter. (Reproduced with permission from Darovic 2002.)

Firstly, the pressure monitoring transducer should be adjusted to the level of the patient's heart. Secondly, the tip of the pulmonary artery catheter should be held at the level of the heart, and the monitor checked to ensure that a pressure of 0 mmHg is recorded (zeroed to atmospheric pressure). Finally, the catheter should be held at the 30 cm mark, and the tip held up to create a vertical fluid column about 30 cm in height, which should produce a pressure equivalent to 22 mmHg. The size (usually 7.5 fg) of the pulmonary artery catheter should be entered into the monitor's data system as well as the volume of injectate being used (Mark 1998, Bridges 2000; Darovic 2002, White 2003).

The position of the patient

Positioning the patient head down will help the catheter float past the tricuspid valve. Tilting the patient on to the right side or placing the head up helps the catheter float out of the right ventricle, remembering that the catheter will tend to float to non-dependent regions as it passes through the heart into the pulmonary artery. Putting the patient in a head up position may reduce the frequency of arrhythmias during catheter insertion. Most catheters will float to the right pulmonary artery (Branthwaite & Bradley 1968, Buchbinder & Gunz 1976, Barash et al 1981, Boyd et al 1983, Darovic 2002, White 2003).

Reliable readings

It has to be remembered that, when using intravascular pressure monitoring systems with fluid-filled catheters, tubing and mechanical transducers are inevitably subject to waveform distortions and pressure values. Many factors contribute to this. For example, blood clots, air bubbles and compliant tubing that is soft will all affect the waveform by damping it and obscuring the detail. Some pressure signals are poorly displayed on the monitor because of the limitations of the monitoring system itself, in that pressure signals with components that are of a high frequency (known as overshoot or ringing or resonance) are displayed as artifact (Mark 1998). It is also worth remembering that normal physiologic pressure waves tend to be more rounded. In contrast, artifactual pressure waves are much sharper in appearance.

In the case of pulmonary artery catheters, as with all other catheters, all lumens should be kept free of air and clots that can affect the quality of the generated waveforms. This is particularly true of the pulmonary artery catheter because it is a much longer catheter. In addition, the catheter is passed through the heart and is affected by its action, displayed as artifact on the screen (Mark 1998, Darovic 2002, White, 2003).

Characteristic pulmonary artery pressure waveforms are displayed once the pulmonary artery catheter is floated into its correct position. Firstly, the pulmonary artery catheter is advanced through the pulmonary artery introducer until the tip of the catheter is in the right atria. The pressure recorded is the central venous or right atrial pressure. This waveform has characteristic a-, c- and v-waves, and a low mean pressure value. With the catheter tip in the right atria, the balloon is inflated with 1.5 ml of air. The pulmonary artery catheter is then advanced until it passes through the tricuspid valve into the right ventricle. At this point, right ventricular pressure can be visualized. The right ventricular pressure waveform can be recognized by the significant increase in systolic pressure and the low diastolic pressure that is similar to right atrial pressure. Early on in diastole, the right ventricular pressure falls to the minimum and then rises during diastole as the right ventricle fills. In order to estimate right ventricular end-diastolic pressure, the electrocardiogram (ECG) R-wave is used as a marker. Having said that, right ventricular pressure does approximate the mean right atrial pressure. This is because right ventricular end-diastolic pressure (RVEDP) is affected by atrial contraction at the end of diastole. As a result, RVEDP is reflected more accurately by the peak of the a-wave (Prentice & Ahrens 2001, White 2003).

As the pulmonary artery catheter passes through the heart from the right ventricle, it floats across the pulmonary valve and into the main pulmonary artery. While it is moving through the right ventricle, arrhythmias are common, as the catheter hits the infundibulum of the right ventricle, particularly causing premature ventricular contractions. It is worth noting that patients may be aware of these arrhythmias, if they occur, and may report unpleasant symptoms. These should subside as the catheter moves out of the right ventricle. The pulmonary artery systolic pressure at this

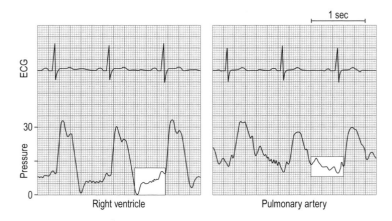

Fig 6.3 The diastolic waveform shape helps distinguish right ventricular from pulmonary artery pressure (shaded areas). During diastole, right ventricular pressure increases as the ventricle fills, while pulmonary artery pressure decreases as blood flows toward the left atrium. (Reproduced with permission from Mark 1998.)

Quiz 6.1

1. *Should the pulmonary artery pressure be higher or lower than the right ventricular systolic pressure?*

2. *What are the three waves of the wedged pulmonary artery trace?*

point should be close to ventricular systolic pressure. However, the pulmonary artery diastolic pressure is generally higher than right ventricular diastolic pressure. This diastolic pressure change helps confirm that the catheter has passed into the pulmonary artery. However, if digital values only are considered, it can be difficult to differentiate between right ventricular pressure and pulmonary artery pressure. By looking at the two waveforms (Figure 6.3), it can be seen that the right ventricular pressure rises during diastole as the blood flows through the open tricuspid value into the right ventricle (Mark 1998, Darovic 2002).

As the pulmonary artery catheter reaches the wedge position, the waveform shape changes and the pulmonary artery wedge pressure looks very much like left atrial pressure with a-, c- and v-waves. It should be noted that the mean pulmonary artery wedge pressure is always less than the mean pulmonary artery pressure, otherwise blood would not be flowing in the right direction (O'Quin & Marini 1983, White, 2003).

Thermodilution

The pulmonary artery catheter estimates cardiac output by use of a thermodilution technique. (The thermodilution cardiac output equation is shown in Appendix 3.) The signal-to-noise ratio, accuracy and precision are greater, the colder the injectate. Having said that, 10 ml of injectate at room temperature will provide an acceptable measurement. In situations where volume overload is a concern, smaller volumes of injectate can be used without significantly affecting the results. It is worth noting that ice-cold injectate has been associated with bradycardia. In order to avoid error owing to variable injectate volumes, it is necessary to be careful when filling syringes. Measurements should be made in the same phase of respiration because it affects cardiac output as well as pulmonary artery blood temperature. Having said that, it is difficult to synchronize injection with respiration. Generally, three evenly spaced measurements with a variation of <10% between measurements

---

Quiz 6.2

1. Do you know what can be done to the patient to aid flotation of the catheter?

2. Do you know when bolus cardiac output readings should be taken in the respiratory cycle?

should give an accurate estimation of cardiac output (Robin 1985, 1988, Roizen et al 1993, Mark 1998, Polanczyk et al 2001, Darovic 2002, White 2003).

Catheter placement

These distances are a rough guide only but, if the pulmonary artery catheter has been inserted through a right jugular vein puncture site, the right atria should be reached when the catheter is inserted 20 cm, the right ventricle at 30–35 cm, the pulmonary artery at 40–45 cm and the wedge position at 50 cm. If other sites have been chosen, additional distance is required. The waveforms should be monitored throughout catheter placement and catheter position confirmed with a chest x-ray (Boyd et al 1983, Bernard et al 2000; White 2003).

Waveform morphologies

The only way to distinguish an artifact from a reliable waveform is through familiarity with the appearance of the normal waveform. For example, the pulmonary artery waveform has a systolic upstroke that is steep, a systolic peak, and a dicrotic notch, followed by a diastolic runoff. The wedge trace on the other hand has a- and v-waves, which can be small. Additional pressure waves that do not follow

Quiz 6.3

1. *From a right jugular vein puncture site, how many centimeters is it to the pulmonary artery?*

2. *What checks should be made to the pulmonary artery catheter prior to insertion?*

a recognizable pattern are often created simply by all the mechanical actions of the heart and heart valves (Mark 1998, Darovic 2002, White 2003).

Continuous pulmonary artery catheter cardiac output

As already discussed, the measurement of cardiac output intermittently involves the use of a pulmonary artery catheter and the bolus thermodilution technique. In contrast, as an alternative to the use of cold thermodilution, the Vigilance monitor is also able to introduce small pulses of energy into the blood continuously, via a product specific pulmonary artery catheter. The monitor then records the temperature of the blood. This enables the Vigilance monitor to compute the cardiac output by using a 'conservation of heat' equation (Boldt et al 1994, Darovic 2002).

The indicator curves are obtained from the temperature waveforms and the energy input, using a cross-correlation technique. A curve is plotted by the monitor that represents the decrease in blood temperature over time. These data are then integrated, based on the Stewart and Hamilton indicator dilution equation (Newman et al 1951). The numeric display (in liters per minute) represents the calculated area beneath the thermodilution curve. The Vigilance monitor is able to perform the calibration process itself, eliminating not only a calibration procedure and the time involved, but also operator error.

When used with an Edwards continuous cardiac output, volumetric and oximetry catheter, the Vigilance monitor (when configured to do so) is able to measure the continuous cardiac output (CCO), continuous end-diastolic volume (EDV) and the mixed venous oxygen saturation ($ScVO_2$).

The end-diastolic volume is measured continuously using the same technology it uses to generate the indicator dilution curves for cardiac output measurement. The patient's heart rate is taken (slaved) from the patient's main hemodynamic monitor ECG signal. The ejection fractions are computed from the continuous average of this heart rate, and the slope of the indicator dilution curve. End-diastolic volume can then be calculated and displayed continuously (without the need for a calibration) from the ejection fraction, heart rate and the cardiac output automatically (Barin et al 2000).

Accuracy of measurements

Inaccurate measurements may be generated for several reasons – physiological, mechanical and electrical. For example, incorrect measurements can result from the incorrect positioning of pulmonary artery catheter, regardless of the type being used, and by flushing cold intravenous fluids repeatedly, even though it is via the infusion lumen of the catheter. Clot formation on the thermistor also affects the catheter's ability to generate accurate data, as does excessive patient movement, variations in the temperature of arterial blood, rapid changes in patients' cardiac output; and the presence of anatomical abnormalities, such as cardiac shunts. Finally, as with many other hemodynamic monitors, the accuracy can be affected by electrical interference from the nearby electrical equipment (Mark 1998, Darovic 2002).

What is wedge pressure?

The pulmonary artery wedge pressure (PAWP) measures the pressure that exists where the blood flow recommences on the venous side of the pulmonary circulation (Figures 6.4 and 6.5). Floating a pulmonary artery catheter until it reaches the wedge position and then 'wedging' it brings about an occlusion of the blood flowing towards a part of the pulmonary vasculature. Between the tip of the pulmonary artery catheter and a point at which the pulmonary veins are not only draining the pulmonary vasculature but also joining other veins still carrying blood towards the left atrium, blood flow stops. This creates a non-flowing column of blood between the pulmonary artery catheter tip (which is wedged) and a bifurcation in the pulmonary veins near to the left atrium (O'Quin & Marini 1983, Mark 1998, Darovic 2002, Pinsky 2003a).

The pulmonary artery wedge pressure is a substitute for left atrial pressure and has very similar waveform components. For example, in the wedge pressure waveform, a- and v-waves (rises in atrial pressure) and the x- and y-descents (falls in atrial pressure) can be identified. Because of the existence of the pulmonary vascular bed between the left atrium and the pulmonary artery catheter tip, the pulmonary wedge pressure is, by an average of 160 ms, a delayed measurement of

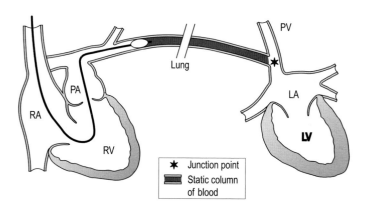

Fig 6.4 Pulmonary artery wedge pressure measurement. The wedged catheter creates a static column of blood connecting the tip of the catheter to a point where the flow resumes in the pulmonary veins near the left atrium. LV, left ventricle; PA, pulmonary artery; RA, right atrium; RV, right ventricle. (Reproduced with permission from Mark 1998.)

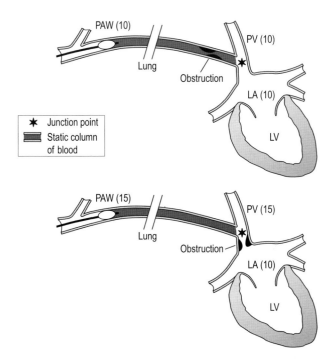

Fig 6.5 Pulmonary veno-occlusive disease. If the flow is obstructed or occluded for some reason, a pressure gradient will be created, resulting in a higher pulmonary artery wedge (PAW) pressure and, therefore, an overestimation of left ventricular end-diastolic pressure. LA, left atrium; LV, left ventricle; PV, pulmonary veins. (Reproduced with permission from Mark 1998.)

the left atrial pressure. This is because it takes time for the left atrial pressure trace to pass through the pulmonary veins, capillaries, arterioles and arteries. Therefore, the a-wave of the wedge pressure waveform follows the R-wave on the ECG during early ventricular contraction (systole), when, in fact, end-diastolic pressure is as a result of atrial contraction. Appreciating this time delay allows accurate waveform interpretation (Pinsky 2003a).

As an alternative to the recording of the pulmonary artery wedge pressure by inflation of the balloon, a wedge pressure can be obtained. This is done by simply advancing the catheter, with the balloon deflated, into a smaller distal branch of the pulmonary artery, allowing indirect measurement of left atrial pressure, thereby reducing the amount of pulmonary vasculature, resulting in less delay and damping of the left atrial pressure waveform (O'Quin & Marini 1983, Mark 1998, Ivanov et al 2000, Darovic 2002, Pinsky 2003b).

It must be remembered that the pulmonary artery wedge pressure is not only a representation of the pressure in the left atrium that is delayed but is also only a reflection of atrial pressure waves that are damped. The degree of damping varies. Having said that, left atrial pressure waves stand out, and there may be a significant underestimation of pressure peaks and troughs measured as inaccurately high levels in the wedge pressure waveform (Mark 1998, Darovic 2002, Pinsky 2003b, White 2003).

In contrast to the central venous pressure waveform, which has three pressure peaks, the pulmonary artery wedge pressure waveform has only two pressure rises that are easy to identify, the a- and v-waves. The c-wave is hard to identify in a normal wedge waveform. This is because, firstly, the a- and c-waves are ordinarily not as well defined in the left atrium as they are in the right, and, secondly, the period of time between the start of atrial and ventricular contraction (and, therefore, the appearance of the a- and c-waves) is shorter on the left side of the heart than it is on the right. As a result, the left atrial a- and c-waves are on top of each other, and this is often referred to as an a–c-wave. Finally, damping also contributes to identification of only two pressure peaks in this waveform (Mark 1998, Pinsky 2003b, White 2003).

It is worth noting that pulmonary artery wedge pressure and pulmonary artery occlusion pressure mean the same thing.

Quiz 6.4

1. *Do you know how the continuous cardiac output differs from bolus cardiac output estimation?*

2. *Can you say what the pulmonary capillary pressure reveals about the pulmonary circulation?*

However, the hydrostatic pressure that exists in the pulmonary capillaries is a different pressure. This pressure must be greater than the left atrial pressure for the blood to flow into the lungs. Having said that, in general terms, the difference between them is small, although can increase significantly in the presence of increased resistance to blood flow in the pulmonary veins (Mark 1998, Pinsky 2003b).

Overwedging

Overwedging happens when the inflation of the pulmonary artery catheter balloon causes the tip of the catheter to become obstructed. Generally, it is caused by the migration of the catheter, forcing the catheter tip up against the wall of the pulmonary artery. Readings obtained are of the gradual rise in pressure that has been produced as a result of the flush system. This pressure continues to rise because the opening is obstructed, until the catheter moves away from the vessel wall. An overwedged pressure waveform is easy to identify. Firstly, it does not pulsate. Secondly, the pressures seen are significantly higher than the pulmonary artery diastolic pressure. The pressure will cease to rise once the balloon is deflated. In order for the catheter to wedge, it has to float a small distance forward, over one or two cardiac cycles. If the catheter wedges before the balloon has been fully inflated, it is likely that the catheter is not in the correct position and has probably floated into a smaller branch of the pulmonary artery. In this situation, the safest thing to do is to withdraw the catheter back somewhat, because otherwise trauma or downstream damage can occur. In addition, the catheter can overwedge itself, without the balloon being inflated at all. This often happens in mechanically ventilated patients (O'Quin & Marini 1983, Mark 1998, Darovic 2002, Pinsky 2003a).

Measurements calculated from the pulmonary artery catheter

In addition to the estimation of cardiac output, the pulmonary artery catheter also provides several calculated values that are thought to be useful clinically. It is worth noting that many of the alternative technologies that estimate cardiac output also derive these values.

Systemic vascular resistance (SVR)

Resistance is the relationship of pressure to flow as determined with reference to Ohm's law. This value is a representation of afterload, the amount of resistance the left ventricle must overcome to eject blood into the aorta (Lake et al 2001).

$$\text{Resistance} = \frac{\text{Mean pressure across the vascular bed}}{\text{Blood flow}}$$

Therefore

$$\text{SVR} = \frac{(\text{MAP} - \text{RAP}) \times 79.96}{\text{CO}}$$

where MAP is mean arterial pressure, RAP is right atrial pressure, CO is cardiac output, and 79.96 is the factor required to convert millimeters of mercury and liters per minute into a resistance measurement.

Since resistance relates pressure to flow, pressure is calculated by measuring the gradient between the proximal (mean arterial) and distal (CVP) ends of the cardiovascular system. It is then divided by the cardiac output to take account of blood flow. SVR reflects an average of all the vascular beds; regional differences are not reflected in this (Darovic 2002).

Pulmonary vascular resistance (PVR)

Pulmonary vascular resistance reflects the resistance to blood flow in the pulmonary circulation. In healthy adults, the pulmonary circulation is usually more compliant than the systemic circulation, so values are lower. The resistance offered by the pulmonary bed is usually one-sixth of that offered by the systemic bed (Mark 1998).

$$\text{Resistance} = \frac{\text{Mean pressure across pulmonary bed}}{\text{Blood flow}}$$

Therefore

$$\text{PVR} = \frac{(\text{MPAP} - \text{PAWP}) \times 79.96}{\text{CO}}$$

where MPAP is mean pulmonary artery pressure, PAWP is pulmonary artery wedge pressure, and 79.96 is the factor required to convert millimeters of mercury and liters per minute into a resistance measurement.

Stroke volume (SV) and stroke volume index (SVI)

These values are not measured but are derived by the previous parameters. Stroke volume is the amount of blood pumped by the ventricle in one contraction. It indicates the contractility state of the heart, and is related to myocardial fiber function and ventricle size. During diastole, the ventricles fill to 120–130 ml (ventricular end-diastolic volume). During systole, 70–80 ml of blood is ejected, accounting for a normal 60% ejection fraction (Seeley 2000).

$$\text{Stroke volume} = \frac{\text{Blood flow}}{\text{Heart rate}} \times 100 \, \text{ml}$$

Therefore

$$SV = \frac{CO}{HR} \times 100 \, \text{ml/l}$$

where CO is cardiac output and HR is heart rate.

Left or right cardiac work index (LCWI/RCWI)

This assesses the amount of work the left or right ventricle performs each minute when ejecting blood. An abnormal value can reflect alterations in either pressure or flow (Mark 1998). It is calculated by:

$$\text{Work} = \frac{\text{Pressure generated} \times \text{volume of blood pumped/min}}{\text{Body surface area}}$$

Therefore:

$$LCWI = \frac{MAP \times SV \times 0.0136}{BSA}$$

$$RCWI = \frac{MPAP \times SV \times 0.0136}{BSA}$$

where MPAP is mean pulmonary artery pressure, BSA is body surface area, and 0.0136 is the factor required to convert millimeters of mercury and liters per minute to a measurement of work.

Note that, for the left side of the heart, the work is calculated by incorporating the mean arterial pressure into the calculation. This is because it is the mean arterial pressure that the heart is working against. On the other hand, for the right side of the heart, the work is against the mean pulmonary artery pressure (Darovic 2002).

Left or right ventricular stroke work index (LVSWI/RVSWI)

This value reflects the amount of work the left or right ventricle undertakes with each beat when ejecting blood. It is calculated by:

$$\text{Work} = \frac{\text{Pressure generated} \times \text{volume of blood pumped}/\text{min}}{\text{Body surface area}}$$

Therefore:

$$\text{LVSWI} = \frac{\text{MAP} \times \text{SV} \times 0.0136}{\text{BSA}}$$

$$\text{RVSWI} = \frac{\text{MPAP} \times \text{SV} \times 0.0136}{\text{BSA}}$$

where 0.0136 is the factor required to convert millimeters of mercury and liters per minute to a measurement of work.

Note that, for the left side of the heart, the work is calculated by incorporating the mean arterial pressure into the calculation. This is because it is the mean arterial pressure that the heart is working against. On the other hand, for the right side of the heart, the work is against the mean pulmonary artery pressure (Mark 1998).

Venous oxygen saturation (SvO$_2$)

A sample of mixed venous blood can be taken from the pulmonary artery catheter and the venous oxygen saturation calculated. Venous oxygen saturation describes the relationship between oxygen delivery and oxygen consumption. Venous oxygen saturation varies directly with cardiac output, hemoglobin and venous oxygen saturation, and inversely with oxygen consumption. A normal venous oxygen saturation does not ensure a normal metabolic state, but suggests that it is either normal or compensated.

Oxygen extraction =

$$\frac{\text{Saturation of arterial blood} - \text{oxygen consumption}}{\text{flow} \times 1.38 \times \text{hemoglobin}}$$

Therefore:

$$SvO_2 = \frac{SaO_2 - VO_2}{CO \times 13.8 \times [Hb]}$$

where SaO_2 is saturation of arterial blood, VO_2 is oxygen consumption, HB is hemoglobin, and 13.8 is the combining power of oxygen to hemoglobin.

Another type of pulmonary artery catheter available is the fiberoptic pulmonary artery catheter. This catheter is able to measure true central venous oxygen saturation ($ScVO_2$) by sampling from the pulmonary artery (Darovic 2002, White 2003).

Monitoring the oxygen content of venous blood

It is important to differentiate straight away the difference between the oxygen content of venous blood and the oxygen content of mixed venous blood. If the blood is sampled from the central venous circulation, the right atrium or superior vena cava, for example, this is the venous oxygen saturation (or SvO_2) and is more reflective of peripheral venous oxygen saturations. If, however, the sample is taken from the pulmonary artery, this is the mixed venous oxygen saturation (or $ScVO_2$) and is more reflective of the central venous oxygen saturation, in that the blood has been mixed with the venous blood draining into the right atrium from the coronary vein. This is important because it reflects myocardial oxygen consumption (Edwards 1990, 1991, Edwards & Mayall 1998, Rivers et al 2001).

Samples taken from the pulmonary artery are thought to be of particular value because of their accuracy as a 'true' mixed venous sample of the patient's blood, differing considerably in the oxygen content of blood taken from the superior vena cava or right atria (Dongre et al 1977, Rivers et al 2001). In the case of a patient in whom the insertion of a pulmonary artery catheter is not possible or practical, a venous oxygen saturation that has been taken from the central line can be measured and used as a trend value. Venous admixture, oxygen delivery and utilization can be calculated (along with other measurements) once the hemoglobin and mixed venous blood samples have been analysed in a blood gas machine (Rivers et al 2001). The determinants of $ScVO_2$ can then be used in the calculation using a modified Fick equation (see Appendix 3).

Errors in the measurement of $ScVO_2$

Under certain conditions, it is possible that specimens of blood taken from the pulmonary artery may not reflect true mixed venous oxygen saturation (Gawlinski 1998). For example, if the pulmonary artery catheter has been wedged at the time of sampling, the oxygen content will reflect either left atrial blood or alveolar capillary blood, depending where the catheter is wedging. The existence of an intracardiac shunt (left or right), as occurs with ventricular septal defects, the oxygen saturation of pulmonary arterial blood will be higher. This is because the mixed venous sample becomes 'arterialized' as it passes through the right ventricular cavity (Birman et al 1984, Cernaianu & Nelson 1993, Gawlinski 1998).

It is worth noting that significant measurement errors in the calculation of derived values can occur, particularly in the venous sample, owing to the shape of the hemoglobin oxygen dissociation curve (i.e. its sigmoid or 'S' shape). In an average individual (70 kg) with a normal metabolic rate, an error in the venous sample measurement of a pH (0.05), or PO_2 (2 mmHg), can result in a 10% error in the oxygen consumption calculation (Gawlinski 1998). In addition, patients who require and are receiving supplemental oxygen, generally, have a central venous oxygen saturation that is higher than that of mixed venous oxygen saturation (Rivers et al 2001).

Continuous monitoring of mixed venous oxygen saturation (ScVO₂)

As already discussed, the $ScVO_2$ is dependent on several variables (hemoglobin, cardiac output, arterial saturation or tissue oxygen). It is not a very specific indicator of the patient's condition because of this, but it does provide a piece of the jigsaw that might help with the overall picture clinically. Having said that, changes in the patient's body demands can result in changes in the mixed venous saturation (Baele et al 1982, Enger & Holm 1990, White 1991).

Quiz 6.5

1. Do you know what systemic vascular resistance is used as a guide to?

2. Can you say what SvO_2 is used to measure?

Both the mortality and morbidity of critically ill patients are known to improve when oxygen delivery (DO_2) and consumption (VO_2) are maintained at an optimum level (Wilson et al 1999). Patients who have normal vital signs but who are critically ill have been demonstrated to have inadequate oxygen delivery (Hassan et al 1989). The continuous monitoring of mixed central venous oxygen saturation allows the total tissue balance of oxygen to be assessed from moment to moment. Mixed venous saturation measurements can be obtained oximetrically, if fiberoptic catheters (Edwards) and appropriate monitors are used (Vigilance). These allow the continuous monitoring of mixed venous saturation ($ScVO_2$), as well as the continuous monitoring of oxygen delivery and oxygen consumption.

In the case of patients at risk of low cardiac output states and those with advanced heart failure, the monitoring of mixed venous oxygen saturation using an oximetric pulmonary artery catheter can be useful as an early indicator of the development of these complications. The advantages of using continuous $ScVO_2$ monitoring, as apposed to intermittent measurements, are that the data are available continuously and, when using continuous cardiac output monitoring, without the need for fluid administration. (This is required for bolus cardiac output with the pulmonary artery catheter and with the PiCCOplus system, which will be discussed later in the chapter.) These advantages can be important, particularly in patients who have pre-existing advanced heart failure or when the patient's ejection fraction is known to be low. Although it is a dependent variable, the $ScVO_2$ can be used as a guide in the determination of trends in tissue oxygenation, after nursing and medical therapies, particularly when used in conjunction with other hemodynamic parameters (Nelson 1986, Hassan et al 1987, Kyff et al 1989, Halfman & Noll 1990,

Noll & Fountain 1990, Pond et al 1992, Scuderi et al 1994, Haller et al 1995, Howard et al 1999, White 2003).

Cardiac output using the Fick method

Application of the Fick principle to oxygen uptake in the lungs can be used to measure cardiac output. This method has traditionally been considered to be the 'gold standard' of cardiac output measurement. However, the preconditions for accurate measurement of cardiac output using the oxygen Fick method are not met in most patients in intensive care units (Lake et al 2001, Darovic 2002, Pittman & Gupta 2003).

Fick proposed that the uptake of oxygen in the lungs is transferred to the blood entirely. This was the first method to estimate cardiac output. Therefore, the cardiac output can be calculated (see Appendix 3) as the ratio between oxygen consumption (VO_2) and the arteriovenous difference in oxygen ($AVDO_2$).

When the patient's hemodynamic status is stable enough to allow consistent diffusion of gas during the mean transit time of blood through the lungs, the estimation is accurate. Having said that, for several reasons, this technique is often not applicable in the critically ill patient. This is essentially because critically ill patients tend to require high levels of oxygen and extreme techniques in order to ventilate them, and often have an unstable hemodynamic status (Pinsky 2003a).

Devices that measure oxygen consumption using indirect calorimetry can be used (with a number of limitations) to calculate cardiac output. For example, both central venous and arterial catheters are required in order to sample mixed venous and arterial blood, and thus compute the arterio-venous oxygen difference. However, this method cannot be used in patients ventilated with a fractional inspired oxygen (FiO_2) greater than 60% because the oxygen sensors are less accurate at these levels.

The Fick principle may be applied to any gas that diffuses through the lungs. This includes carbon dioxide. Monitors utilizing this principle are based its application to carbon dioxide in order to estimate cardiac output non-invasively. Having said that, the patient has to be mechanically venti-lated. The monitor involves the patient partially rebreath-ing intermittently through a disposable rebreathing loop, which is specific to the product. The monitor comprises a carbon dioxide sensor (infrared) and a disposable airflow sensor for carbon dioxide, which works by the absorption of the infrared light and a pulse oximeter. The oxygen con-sumption is calculated from the minute ventilation and carbon dioxide content. The arterial carbon dioxide content ($CaCO_2$) is estimated from the end-tidal carbon dioxide ($etCO_2$). Adjustments have to be made for the degree of dead-space ventilation and for the slope of the carbon dioxide dissociation curve.

Obviously, the partial rebreathing reduces the elimination of carbon dioxide and so increases $etCO_2$. The need for central venous access is unnecessary with this technology because normal and rebreathing conditions allow the omis-sion of the venous carbon dioxide content ($CvCO_2$). It is assumed that cardiac output remains unchanged under normal and under rebreathing conditions. By subtracting both the normal and the rebreathing ratios, a differential Fick equation is then obtained (Darovic 2002).

As carbon dioxide quickly diffuses in blood (22 times more quickly than oxygen), it is assumed that the venous carbon dioxide content will not change between normal and rebreathing conditions. This means that the venous content is removed from the equation (Edwards 1998). The carbon dioxide dissociation curve represents the relationship between volumes of carbon dioxide, which are then used to calculate the carbon dioxide content, as well as its partial pressure. Between 15 and 70 mmHg of partial pressure of carbon dioxide, the relationship is considered to be linear (Darovic 2002).

Changes in oxygen consumption and end-tidal carbon dioxide only reflect the flow of blood that takes part in gas exchange. In the case of an intrapulmonary shunt, estimation of cardiac output using the non-invasive cardiac output (NICO) monitor device (which we will return to later in this section) can be affected. The monitor is able to take this into account by estimating the shunting fraction. It does this by using the fraction of inspired oxygen combined with a measured peripheral oxygen saturation of hemoglobin and the arterial oxygen tension (using Nunn's iso-shunt tables). Obviously, an arterial blood gas reading needs to be taken to do this. Poor hemodynamic stability and an increased intrapulmonary shunt are common in most critically ill patients. As both these factors can affect the accuracy of cardiac output estimated by the NICO monitor, its use in this group of patients may be limited. Although beyond the scope of this book, the NICO monitor does provide interesting respiratory data that may have a role in the management of the critically ill patient.

It is important to note that the patient must be under fully controlled mechanical ventilation if the NICO monitor is to be used. In addition, arterial blood samples are required to enter arterial oxygen tension values for shunt estimation, which somewhat tempers the non-invasive nature of this technique.

Non-invasive cardiac output monitor

Non-invasive cardiac output is based on the Fick method, which is the standard reference technique used to evaluate other means of determining cardiac output. The conventional Fick method is based on the principle that oxygen consumption is proportional to the rate of blood pumped by the heart through the lungs, and it can be measured by monitoring gas exchange and invasively sampling blood gases. NICO uses the Fick principle applied to carbon dioxide produced by the body, and eliminated through gas exchange in the lungs.

The NICO system is completely non-invasive and easy to use, merely requiring placement of the NICO sensor between the endotracheal tube and the breathing circuit Y piece. NICO automatically cycles through brief periods of partial rebreathing, providing a cardiac output.

Thoracic electrical bioimpedance monitoring

Since this time, several improvements have been made. In 1982, the BioMed non-invasive continuous cardiac output monitor was marketed (Imhoff et al 2000). The BioMed, using an analog-based processing technique, calculated cardiac output from the observed heart rate and the use of equations that are based on healthy volunteers. Since its initial development, the BioMed has been improved and now replaced by the BioZ (Cardiodynamics, San Diego, CA, USA).

A small amplitude of 0.2–0.4 mA alternating current at 40 kHz is introduced by electrodes in order to create an electrical field, which passes across the thorax from the base of the neck to the junction of the xiphisternum (Figure 6.6). The electrical signal predominantly travels down the aorta, as opposed to travelling through the alveoli, which are air filled. Throughout the cardiac cycle, the changes in aortic flow correlate with changes in impedance. The changes in impedance then appear on the monitor as a series of rises and falls in impedance, and correlate to the cardiac cycle (Figure 6.7; Critchley 1998, Genoni et al 1998).

Berstein made several changes to the original model, including correcting the original idea of the thorax as a cylinder and mathematically representing the thorax as a truncated cone. As a result, the software was modified by altering the averaging of the impedance waveforms.

The impedance (dZ/dt) waveforms have to be looked at and assessed in order to establish their accuracy. Some of the

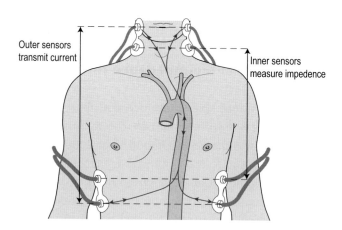

Fig 6.6 Diagram indicating the correct placement of special electrodes for measuring voltage changes across the thorax. (Reproduced with permission from Darovic 2002.)

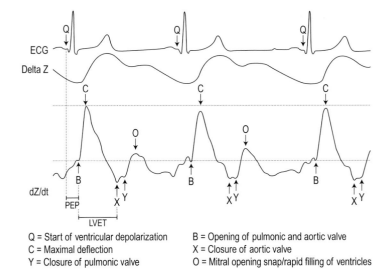

Q = Start of ventricular depolarization
C = Maximal deflection
Y = Closure of pulmonic valve

B = Opening of pulmonic and aortic valve
X = Closure of aortic valve
O = Mitral opening snap/rapid filling of ventricles

Fig 6.7 Diagram of the impedance waveform in relation to the normal electrocardiogram. (Reproduced with permission from Darovic 2002.)

Quiz 6.6

1. What is a thoracic electrical bioimpedance monitor?

2. Can you identify the parameters the thoracic electrical bioimpedance monitor measures?

earlier impedance models had simple 'look up' tables, averaging techniques to detect impedance thresholds. The user interfaces were also complicated. Transient information was frequently lost because of interference with the frequency and amplitude, and the process of impedance determination (Darovic 2002).

In patients who have increasing lung fluid during systole, electrical signals bypass aortic flow and can result in inaccurate values being generated. This is because of the low signal to noise ratios. For example, significant differences between bioimpedance and thermodilution calculations have been seen in patients with pleural effusions, pulmonary edema, severe congestive heart failure, severe pneumonia and hemothorax (Darovic 2002). In each of these conditions, the distortions in the electrical field has been due to abnormal fluid and electrolytes being present in the thorax, allowing the electrical signal to bypass the source of impedance changes, which is aortic blood flow (Darovic 2002).

Patients who have a heart rate greater than 140 beats per minute have a total blood flow down the aorta during systole that is much less than that in patients with a normal heart rate. This results in an estimated cardiac output using impedance that may be much lower that its actual value (Imhoff et al 2000).

The esophageal Doppler monitor

History

Originally, the Doppler as a principle was suggested by Christian Johanne Doppler (1803–1853), who was a mathematician and assistant to the professor of mathematics at the Bohemia University of Prague. In 1845, the Doppler theory was confirmed by using a steam train and musicians (Buys Ballot 1817–1890). Horn players with perfect pitch were on the train playing a constant note and pitch-perfect listeners stood by the track of the Utrecht railway, Amsterdam, recording what they heard as the train approached and the note as it went away.

Principle

If an ultrasound beam is directed at a column of blood flowing down it, there will be a shift in frequency in the reflected sound (brought about by the flow of red blood cells in the descending aorta, which lies close and parallel). This is known as the Doppler shift. The degree, or magnitude, of the Doppler shift in frequency and angle of incidence is directly proportional to the speed (velocity) of blood flow. This is the Doppler principle (Singer & Bennett 1991, Singer et al 1991, Valtier et al 1998, DiCorte et al 2000).

It is presumed that all red blood cells move at approximately the same velocity. This problem has been solved by the manufacturers of Doppler probes and monitors by either having an echo transducer in the probe itself to measure the diameter of the aorta instantaneously (HemoSonic, Arrow), or by the use of normograms (CardioQ, Deltex Medical Ltd; and Waki, Atys Medical), to approximate the cross-sectional area of the descending aorta. Stroke volume can be calculated by taking the average blood velocity during an ejection phase of the cardiac cycle and multiplying it by the stroke distance (ejection time) and the cross-sectional area of the descending aorta through which blood flows (Buhre et al 1993, Darmon et al 1994, Mathews & Nevin 1998, Perrino et al 1998, Oates 2001, Darovic 2002).

As a tool for measuring hemodynamics, the esophageal Doppler method of measuring cardiac output has undergone several developments since its first introduction into critical care units. Mervyn Singer (London, England) and his colleagues have been instrumental in the past and present stage of development of the Cardiac Q monitor and probe (Deltex Medical, Chichester, UK). Singer and colleagues have described an esophageal Doppler system with a new continuous-wave (Singer & Bennett 1991). This system has been referred to by several names – ODM-1, the ODM-2 and the Cardiac Q (Deltex Medical, Chichester, UK) – and has passed through several stages of development. In the first instance, the system was used to look at the cardiac output measured by the thermodilution method and compare the measurements with trends in aortic blood flow (Oates, 2001; Darovic, 2002; Seoul et al, 2003).

However, Singer went on to estimate total left ventricular cardiac output by developing a normogram (referred to earlier). This normogram is based on the patient's height, weight and age, without the need for additional hemodynamic measurements. The use of the normogram enables the corrected estimate of total left ventricular cardiac output to be translated into Doppler values for the descending aorta. The strong correlation in the cardiac output measurements obtained allowed an important conclusion to be drawn. This was that, despite changes in arterial blood pressure, cardiac output and body temperature (although these were not formally examined), and the flow of blood down the descending thoracic aorta were the same (fixed and in proportion) as the total left ventricular cardiac output (Singer & Bennett 1991, Oates 2001). Estimating aortic diameter is recognized as a potential source of error in that the error margin can easily be increased in the subsequent calculation of the cross-sectional area of the aorta. This is because the squared radius is used in the calculation. A 2 mm error in a 25 mm aortic diameter equates to a 16% error in total (Singer & Bennett 1991, Lefrant et al 1998, Oates 2001).

Insertion of a Doppler probe

Esophageal Doppler is a simple technique, and most users acknowledge that it is fairly easy to achieve adequate probe positioning and to obtain reproducible results. A thin, flexible, silicone probe of approximately 6 mm diameter is passed down the patient's esophagus. The probes are for single person use, and are specific for the purpose and the monitor being used. The patient should ideally be lightly sedated and ventilated in order to tolerate an oral probe. However, some patients may tolerate the probe without sedation, although frequent movement interferes with the signal. The probe is then advanced to a position where it is located along side the descending aorta (Figure 6.8). The other end of the probe is then connected to the monitoring system via a transducing cable. It should be noted that the ultrasound beam itself is harmless to the patient (Darovic 2002).

Accurate measurement of cardiac output depends on the correct positioning of the probe. This is an important point. Using the depth markings on the probe as a guide, the probe is then advanced gently until the tip is located approximately at the mid-thoracic level. It can then be rotated so that the transducer faces the aorta (Darovic 2002). A 4 MHz continuous or 5 MHz pulsed wave transducer is used, according to the type of device. Once the characteristic waveform (descending aortic trace) is visualized, it can be optimized by the slow rotation and alteration of the depth of insertion, to generate a clear audible signal with the highest possible peak velocity (Schmid et al 1993, Marik et al 1997, Poelaert et al 1999, Pittman & Gupta 2003). The probe can then be left in place and its depth

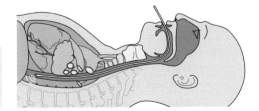

Fig 6.8 Positioning of the esophageal probe. (Reproduced with permission from Shoemaker et al 2002.)

noted. The gain setting can be altered in order to obtain the best contour of the aortic velocity waveform (Darovic 2002).

Knowledge of the angle at which the blood is flowing, and optimal alignment between this blood flow and the Doppler beam is crucial, if accurate velocity measurements are to be obtained. This can be judged when the brightest signal is visualized (CardioQ, Deltex Medical Ltd, Chichester, UK; Waki, Atys Medical, Soucieu en Jarrest, France) or if on M-mode echocardiography (HemoSonic, Arrow International, Reading, PA, USA), the aortic walls are well defined. Because the angle of the esophagus and aorta are ordinarily parallel in the thorax, it is presumed that this angle is the same for the flow of blood and Doppler beam, transducer and probe. This is between 45° and 60° depending on the type of probe used. Errors in the theoretical and true angle can be significant (Oates 2001).

One of the biggest drawbacks of the Doppler system, from experience, is the ease with which the signal necessary to generate accurate data can be lost. Patient movement owing to agitation or nursing and/or medical interventions frequently results in loss of the signal and poorly defined velocity. Oral tubes are generally poorly tolerated in patients who are either minimally or not sedated. These patients tend to move around a great deal. Having said that, the probe can be easily repositioned, once the patient is settled (Oates 2001).

Waveform characteristics

The characteristics of the esophageal Doppler waveform can be used to assist both in the diagnosis and treatment options for patients.

The waveform area (velocity-time or stroke distance) is comparable to the flow of blood passing down the descending aorta, and to the left ventricular stroke volume. The real-time display of a velocity-time waveform is available on most esophageal Doppler monitors (Figure 6.9). In addition to the size of the waveform, additional information can be derived from its shape. It is normal for the peak velocity to decline with increasing age (1% per annum approximately). High or low predicted peak velocity readings outside the normal range (90–120 cm/s in a resting adult) may indicate either a hyperdynamic or hypodynamic state (Oates 2001, Darovic 2002).

The efficiency of left ventricular contractility is reflected in the mean acceleration and peak velocity. Both peak velocity and mean acceleration would be increased in patients receiving positive inotropes (to increase contractility; Figure 6.10). However, in myocardial ischemia or myocardial depression, a low value would be expected (reduced contractility owing to myocardial damage). Peak velocity and

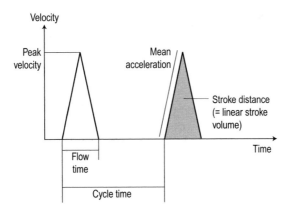

Fig 6.9 Doppler velocity–time waveform. (Reproduced with permission from Shoemaker et al 2002.)

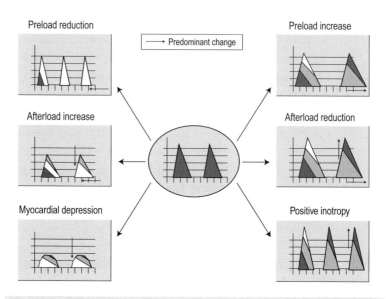

Fig 6.10 Changes in waveform shape with hemodynamic maneuvers. (Reproduced with permission from Shoemaker et al 2002.)

mean acceleration are also affected by changes in preload (to a small degree) and afterload (to a higher degree).

The time intervals of systole and diastole are affected by the heart rate: they are reduced in tachycardia and increased in bradycardia. The base of the esophageal Doppler waveform is the flow-time axis and, as such, is dependent upon the patient's heart rate. Incidentally, it is possible to correct this by using an equation that alters the time interval (Bazett's equation, which divides flow time by the square root of the time cycle). The normal range for this corrected flow time (FTc) is 0.33–0.36 s (in a normal individual). There is an inverse relationship between the corrected flow time and the systemic vascular resistance. For example, if the patient is hypovolemic or hypothermic, a narrow corrected flow-time waveform would be expected. However, in the severely septic patient, when considerable vasodilation occurs, a broad corrected flow time would be consistent with the patient's condition clinically (Singer & Bennett 1991, Darovic 2002).

The esophageal Doppler waveforms (as with all waveforms obtained from hemodynamic monitors) can give some diagnostic clues (in conjunction with other hemodynamic data) to the patient's degree of critical illness (Sinclair and James et al 1997). For example, the ability of the myocardium to contract effectively can be assessed by looking at the height of the waveform and the slope of its upstroke. The systemic vascular resistance, as well as the efficiency of the heart valves (regurgitation), is reflected in the width of the waveform: a small narrow waveform suggests some degree of cardiac or pulmonary obstruction, especially if associated with an increased central venous pressure.

In summary, the esophageal Doppler as a hemodynamic monitor is minimally invasive when compared to other monitors estimating cardiac output. It provides real-time information about emerging trends, although absolute values of cardiac output are not very accurate. The probe is easy to insert, but can be more difficult to position it correctly. However, the online educational support that is available for some esophageal Doppler monitors is of great help. The Doppler probe is affected by the presence of a nasogastric tube and dislodgement by patient movement. In some patients, the insertion of an esophageal probe is

Quiz 6.7

1. *Can you list the advantages and disadvantages of the esophageal Doppler technique?*

2. *Do you know what the principle underpinning this technology is?*

contraindicated (e.g. postesophagectomy patients or patients with an esophageal injury; Darovic 2002).

Pulse contour and pulse power technologies

In November 1951, Newman et al (1951) published an evaluation of the dye dilution method of describing the central circulation. The principle of dye dilution depends on the assumption that the indicator is distributed throughout a central pool of blood as it passes from the venous system, through the heart and lungs, and into the arterial circulation. From the point of view of pulse-power and pulse-contour technologies, some interesting conclusions were arrived at. For example, information could be derived from the shape of the curve and this was governed not only by flow, but also by volume in a central pool. This pool was not made up of a single volume but of a series of volumes, and the size of these could be calculated (Newman et al 1951).

The mechanical features of the arterial system and its relationship to stroke volume result in the aortic pressure waveform. Almost a hundred years ago, the first attempt to use the shape of the arterial pulse curve in order to estimate stroke volume was made. The simplest of the models ('Windkessel' models) that have been proposed since then, is still being utilized today, in principle, although it has been subject to many improvements (Wesseling et al 1993, Pittman & Gupta 2003).

In this first and simple model, the value of the mean arterial pressure for any given blood flow is determined by a single resistance (peripheral resistance), which corresponds to the degree of vasoconstriction in small arteries (arterial tone). However, this model (the two-element 'Windkessel' model) is limited in its ability to reproduce the shape of the aortic pulse curve faithfully. This is because the shape of the curve cannot be explained by the peripheral resistance alone: other components must be included in the model. Adding another factor, a capacitance component, creates a more physiological pulse-pressure wave. The addition of a further factor to represent the features of aortic impedance, allows the creation of a predicted waveform that is very similar to that which the model intends to simulate. The three-element 'Windkessel' model includes an aortic impedance component (Pittman & Gupta 2003).

More complex models take into account the velocity and reflection of the pulse wave. Resistance, compliance and characteristic impedance values are estimated initially from the age and sex of the patient, and from the pressure waveform. These estimates are then refined by a calibration technique in order to obtain the patient's cardiac output (Zollner et al, 2000).

An initial calibration, regardless of the model used, by whichever method, will improve the accuracy of the predicted cardiac output. This is because the calibration provides a reference value for the ratio of mean arterial pressure to the mean systemic flow (peripheral resistance), enabling a more accurate estimate of cardiac output and other parameters representing the mechanical properties of the arterial system. Recalibration is generally performed in accordance with the manufacturer's guidelines, and when a patient's hemodynamic status and/or treatment are changing significantly (Pittman & Gupta 2003).

Pulse contour

Deriving stroke volume from the pulse contour (or shape of the waveform) involves analysis of only the systolic area of the arterial waveform. In order to achieve this, the catheter and transducer used, by necessity, have to be as central and near to the aorta as possible (although not in it). This is to allow for the identification of the dicrotic notch, which denotes the end of systole, and the reflective wave, which can change the systolic area (Godje et al 2002; Pittman & Gupta 2003).

Pulse power

In order to derive the stroke volume from the pulse power (Power of the arterial pulse), the entire arterial pressure waveform is analysed. The volume of blood, the stroke volume, which is forced into the arterial circulation with each systolic ejection, causes the arterial blood pressure to vary around a mean value. The degree of pressure change, the pulse pressure, is related to the amount of stroke volume ejected. However, the compliance of the arterial wall plays an important part. The greater the compliance of the arterial wall, the less the increase in arterial pressure when the stroke volume is ejected during systole. Aortic compliance is not linear. This makes any straightforward approach to using the pulse pressure to estimate aortic compliance difficult. Having said that, it is possible to obtain a total aortic compliance by adding the compliances of the different sections together (Jonas & Tanser 2002b).

Although there is less reflection in the aortic wave than anywhere else in the arterial tree, this relection still has to be taken into account and corrected for. Intrinsically, age (particularly the elderly), velocity, ejection time and flow during systole, and the capacity of the arterial system itself contribute to waveform reflection. From an extrinsic point of view, the properties of the arterial waveform transducing system can also affect the degree of reflection in the waveform (Mark 1998, Godje et al 2000).

The shape and size of the arterial waveform are affected by reflection, and result in the augmentation of the arterial blood pressure. As already implied, the pulse pressure then is the product of the velocity of the pulse wave (ventricular ejection) against a particular resistance and the reflective wave. It follows that, from the aorta to the peripheral arteries, the pulse pressure rises considerably (Mark 1998, Darovic 2002, Zollner et al 2002).

The LiDCOplus™ monitoring system

Following an initial lithium calibration, the monitoring system provides a minimally invasive method of measuring and continuously monitoring cardiac output, oxygen delivery, and other important hemodynamic variables. The LiDCOplus™ (Lithium InDicator Cardiac Output Plus; LiDCO plc, Cambridge, UK) achieves this by analysing the arterial blood pressure waveform from the patient's standard peripheral arterial line. The LiDCOplus™ is suitable for the majority of critically ill patients who require venous and arterial access, and monitoring of their hemodynamic status (Linton et al 1993).

Background

The original indicator dilution technique was based on the principle of the dilution of a known amount of indicator, developed by Stewart-Hamilton. The technique was labor intensive, in that frequent blood analysis was required, and difficult to undertake because of its complexity. A much simpler 'dilution of an indicator' method using lithium as the indicator was initially proposed by Terry O'Brien in 1993 and is the indicator utilized for the calibration of the LiDCOplus™ today (Jonas et al 1999, Garcia-Rodriguez et al 2002).

Arterial waveform into cardiac output

In order to obtain an accurate continuous cardiac output from the analysis of the arterial waveform and calibration, the blood pressure waveform itself has to be transformed. This involves three stages. The first involves the conversion of the arterial waveform into a volume–time waveform. From this it is possible to derive a nominal, or supposed stroke volume, and the duration of the heartbeat. To then obtain an actual stroke volume, the mathematical method of autocorrelation is used. This is the second stage. Auto-correlation derives not only the length of the heartbeat but also the overall effect of the heartbeat, or power factor, which is directly in proportion to the nominal, or supposed stroke volume ejected from the aorta (Pittman & Gupta 2003).

The third stage involves the nominal stroke volume and, therefore, cardiac output, to be derived from an algorithm. This is then converted to the actual stroke volume by the use of lithium as an independent indicator, and a transpulmonary dilution technique, using the LiDCOplus™, to obtain a patient-specific calibration factor (compliance correction of arterial pulse power for a specific patient). It does this by multiplying the nominal stroke volume by the calibration factor derived from the individual patient. The precision of the calibration is very important to obtain accurate data. Although adequate, thermodilution does not have ideal accuracy. The pulmonary artery catheter thermodilution, with its three-bolus technique, is used as the comparison for any other calibration method. Therefore, the accuracy of other methods, in terms of the cardiac output measurement obtained, should be at least equal to, and preferably better than pulmonary artery catheter thermodilution, within a range of ±15% (Pearse et al 2004).

Lithium chloride

The safety of lithium chloride is widely recognized and the maximum dose recommended (0.075–0.3 mmol of lithium chloride per calibration) is just 1/250th of that prescribed to patients requiring therapeutic lithium therapy. It can be seen that the recommended dose would have to be considerably surpassed for it to become in any way toxic to the patient. As a marker, lithium is robust for the measurement of cardiac output using transpulmonary indicator dilution because ordinarily it is not present in the body in any form. Both the injection of the lithium bolus (vein) and detection of it as a marker (artery) can be obtained peripherally, from the cubital vein to the pedal artery (Peruzzi 2000). Before the lithium dose is recirculated, the cardiac output is calculated from the lithium dose and the area beneath the concentration–time curve generated (Linton et al 1993, 1995, 1997). The following equation is used:

$$\text{Cardiac output} = \frac{\text{dose of lithium (mmols)} \times 60}{\text{Area} \times (1 - \text{packed cell volume}) \, (\text{mmols/sec})}$$

Setting up the system

As the LiDCOplus™ does not require the insertion of additional invasive lines (because it only needs those usually already in place in critically ill patients), it takes little time and is simple to set up. The system utilizes the existing fluid-filled arterial line transducer set, adding into the circuit an ion-selective electrode that detects the lithium chloride during the indicator dilution process (Linton et al

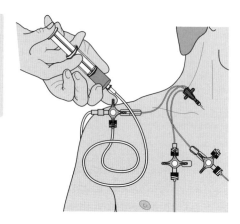

Fig 6.11 A known volume and concentration of lithium are injected into a vein. A central vein is used in this figure, although a peripheral line can also be used and gives the same degree of accuracy.

1998, 2002, Jonas 2001, Jonas et al 2002). The sensor is primed with saline and then attached to the patient (Figure 6.11).

Information is obtained from three sources. Firstly, blood gas parameters, such as the hemoglobin, the saturation of arterial blood, the systolic, diastolic and mean pressures, and the systolic, pulse and stroke volume variations, are obtained from peripheral arterial access. Secondly, an accurate cardiac output is obtained following calibration. Finally, the continuous display of cardiac output and oxygen delivery is made possible from the software from which the LiDCOplus™ monitor is working (Figure 6.12; Jonas & Tanser 2002b).

The accuracy of LiDCOplus™ is not adversely affected by intrinsic or extrinsic factors, for example, the limitations of the arterial transducer system, such as overdamping, or a lower than normal natural frequency (see Chapter 3). It is also unaffected by the presence of pulmonary edema, tricuspid incompetence (regurgitation) or infusions of fluid. In the absence of drift, recalibration is only indicated if the level of drug infusions a patient is receiving that affects

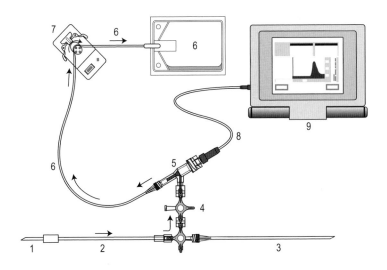

Fig 6.12 Blood moves from the patient's arterial line past the sensor to a collection bag with the aid of a roller pump. This allows the exact level of lithium to be detected by the sensor as it does so.

systemic vascular resistance is greater than the accuracy of the initial calibration itself.

Limitation of the LiDCOplus™

As with most hemodynamic monitoring systems, there are some situations and certain conditions that affect the ability of the system to perform well. There are both intrinsic and extrinsic reasons for this. For example, intrinsically, aortic valve regurgitation, left to right shunts, aorta reconstruction, severe peripheral arterial vasoconstriction or peripheral vascular disease, irregular heart rates, hypothermia and intra-aortic balloon pumps all affect accuracy of the system.

Extrinsically, arterial lines that are severely damped with associated problems involving the catheter site, transducer or pressure line affect accuracy. Changing the primary general monitor being used in conjunction with the LiD-COplus™ following calibration can affect the calibration factor that has been derived.

It is worth noting that the use of lithium as an indicator is contraindicated in pregnant women during the first trimester, in those already receiving lithium therapy and in the presence of some muscle relaxants. However, it is possible to obtain a cardiac output measurement from another source in these circumstances. For example, the cardiac output value can be taken from an esophageal Doppler or pulmonary artery catheter, and entered into the LiD-COplus™. This enables the system to derive stroke volume, and display cardiac output and other variables continuously as described in this section.

Its accuracy, precision and minimally invasive design is making this system a popular tool in the management of the critically ill patient (Linton et al 1997, 2002, Garcia-Rodriguez et al 2002, Jonas & Tanser 2002, Jonas et al 2002). As new invasive lines do not need to be inserted, the system can be set up and managed totally by nurses; this is a very important point.

The Pulsion PiCCOplus™ monitoring system

The Pulsion PiCCOplus™ (Pulse Contour Cardiac Output. Manufactured by Pulsion Medical Systems, Kimal, Middlesex) is a hemodynamic monitoring method that is intended to determine and monitor both cardiopulmonary and circulatory function, utilizing a combination of transpulmonary thermodilution and arterial pulse contour analysis. The PiCCOplus hemodynamic monitoring system is able to derive several parameters, some of which are unique to this device (Lichtwarck-Ascoff et al 1992, Bindels et al 1999, Salukhe & Wyncoll 2002).

From transpulmonary thermodilution (we will return to this calibration technique later), including transpulmonary cardiac output, cardiac function index, intrathoracic blood volume, global diastolic volume, extravascular lung water, pulmonary vascular permeability index and the global ejection fraction are measured or derived (Pfeiffer et al 1994). These parameters will be explained in more detail later in this section. After an initial calibration, pulse contour analysis derives the heart rate, systolic, diastolic and mean arterial pressures, pulse contour cardiac output, stroke volume, systemic vascular resistance, index of left ventricular contractility, and both pulse and stroke volume variations (Bindels et al 1999, 2000).

Principle

The PiCCOplus system works on the principle that, when a known volume and temperature of a thermal indicator (ice-cold saline) is injected into a central vein, both volumetric and thermal dispersal within the pulmonary and cardiac volumes occurs rapidly. The wrong setting of both volume and temperature can result in incorrect cardiac output estimation. The volume distributed is referred to as the intrathoracic volume. Once the arterial thermistor detects the thermal signal, the difference in temperature is detected and a curve is created (Salukhe & Wyncoll 2002). By the application of the Stewart–Hamilton equation, cardiac output is calculated (Hoeft 1995).

Calibration of the PiCCOplus

In order to perform a thermodilution measurement, otherwise referred to as a calibration, the patient requires central venous access (preferably internal jugular or subclavian) and a product-specific arterial line (which has a built-in thermistor). It is worth noting at this point that, if the femoral vein is used for central venous access, the cardiac output readings can be overestimated by up to 75 ml/min (Hoeft 1995).

If the patient already has an arterial line, this can either be left in place or removed, as both blood sampling and the transducing of arterial pressures can be obtained from the product-specific catheter (Figure 6.13). Only disposables and accessories approved by PULSION Medical Systems can be used in conjunction with the PiCCOplus. The site of the arterial access is recommended to be the femoral, brachial or axillary arteries. It is important not to advance the

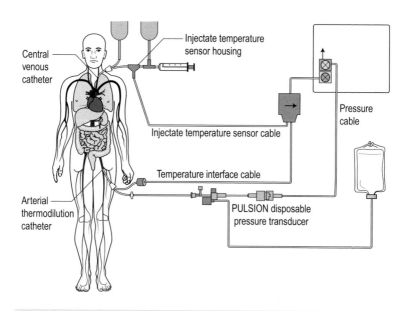

Fig 6.13 A known volume of fluid is injected into a central vein. The temperature of the fluid is detected by a sensor on injection and the temperature change over time is then measured as the blood passes a sensor located at the site of the arterial line.

Quiz 6.8

1. Which parameters do the PiCCOplus and transpulmonary thermodilution system measure?

2. Do you know which arteries have to be used?

Quiz 6.9

1. What does the Fick principle rely upon?

2. What is a PiCCOplus calibration, what is a LiDCO calibration and what do they measure?

catheter into the aorta on insertion (Lichtwarck-Ascoff et al 1992, Bindels et al 1999, Salukhe & Wyncoll 2002).

The indicator, usually ice-cold saline, is injected into the central line rapidly and smoothly (as for the pulmonary artery catheter bolus cardiac output technique) and no other infusions should be switched on or bolus injections given at this point. The temperature of the injectate should be at least 10°C colder than the patient's body temperature. The PiCCOplus advises on the injectate volume to use for a specific patient, depending on body weight and the temperature of the injectate (the greater the body weight, the greater the volume). In addition, the lower the temperature of the injectate, the higher the volume of injectate is required for an accurate estimate of cardiac output. It is worth noting that none of the cold indicator is lost while it is passing through the heart and lungs. This means that the timing of injection of the indicator in relation to the respiratory cycle is not crucial (Salukhe & Wyncoll 2002).

In the stable patient, recalibration is recommended every 8 hours. However, the manufacturers' recommend recalibration may be necessary hourly while the patient is being actively resuscitated. If there are significant changes in the patient's hemodynamic status or the cardiac output is consistently changing in the same direction for more that 15 minutes, recalibration should be performed. It is worth noting that, before the PiCCOplus can be considered calibrated, the arterial waveform and thermodilution curve must be considered to be acceptable from a technical point of view (Kouchoukos et al 1970, Pfeiffer et al 1994, Rödig et al 1999).

The algorithm

The PiCCO algorithm is based on the Stewart–Hamilton method. Following acceptable calibration, pulse-induced contour cardiac output, arterial blood pressure, heart rate, stroke volume, systemic vascular resistance, intrathoracic blood volume, extravascular lung water and cardiac function index are continually quantified and displayed. Several other hemodynamic monitors measure the first five parameters. However, the remaining three parameters are unique to the PiCCOplus and will be considered in detail (Table 6.3).

Intrathoracic blood volume

The thorax has a limited ability to expand. Because of this, the three volumes contained within it, intrathoracic blood volume (ITBV), intrathoracic gas volume and extravascular lung water, change and interact with each other proportionately. It is worth noting that the thorax has a potential fourth compartment that can increase the overall volume of the thoracic cavity (e.g. space-occupying tumours or pleural effusions). The intrathoracic blood volume is composed of the pulmonary blood volume (20%), and the

Table 6.3 Parameters obtained by transpulmonary thermodilution.[a] (Adapted from the PiCCO Instruction Manual)		
Parameter	Absolute (abbreviation and units)	Indexed (abbreviation and units)
Transpulmonary cardiac output	COa (l/min)	CIa (l/min per m²)
Cardiac function index	CFI (l/min)	
Intrathoracic blood volume	ITBV (ml)	ITBVI (ml/m²)
Global end-diastolic volume	GEDV (ml)	GEDI (ml/m²)
Extravascular lung water	EVLW (ml)	EVLWI (ml/kg)
Pulmonary vascular permeability index	PVPI	
Global ejection fraction	GEF (%)	

[a]The parameters above are derived by the PiCCOplus from a central venous injection and transpulmonary detection with a thermodilution catheter. *The application of a pulmonary artery catheter is not necessary.*

global end-diastolic volume of all four chambers of the heart (80%).

Intrathoracic blood volume is calculated by using the mean transit time of the cold injectate and the subsequently derived cardiac output from the thermodilution calibration that has been performed. The relationship between cardiac output and the mean transit time is independent, in that there is no mathematical connection between the two (Sturm 1990, Lichtwarck-Ascoff et al 1992, Bindels et al 1999, Sakka et al 2000, Salukhe & Wyncoll 2002).

Global end-diastolic volume

The global end-diastolic volume (GEDV) is equivalent to the preload of the four heart chambers, because it is the sum of all end-diastolic volumes of both atria and both ventricles. It is determined by the PiCCOplus through the thermodilution technique (Sakka et al 2000).

Extravascular lung water

Extravascular lung water (EVLW) is equal to the intravascular thermal volume minus the estimated intrathoracic blood volume. This is the mean transit time method used by the PiCCOplus. It is possible to subdivide extravascular lung water into three compartments: interstitial fluid, intracellular fluid and intra-alveolar fluid.

The interstitial fluid is the free fluid found in interstitial spaces and is limited in the normal lung. If fluid accumulates owing to a pathological process, these spaces act as a buffer, by taking up this additional fluid. This mechanism protects the integrity of the alveolar–capillary membrane up to a point. If the degree of interstitial edema becomes greater than 10 ml/kg of body weight, these spaces will expand and become separated by the accumulation of fluid (Hoeft 1995). Intracellular fluid is the fluid found in the cells of the lung tissue and represents approximately 40% of the overall fluid content of the lungs. If the cells fail to function normally, a significant amount of fluid can shift into these cells (Sturm 1990). Fluid within the tissues of the lung (intra-alveolar fluid) can increase by up to 300% before the fluid will move into the alveoli (Lichtwarck-Ascoff et al 1992, Bindels et al 1999, Salukhe & Wyncoll 2002).

An approximate estimation of extravascular lung water can be made from the dilution of an indicator (ice-cold fluid) between two points, allowing the calculation of the volume inbetween them. The difference between the two volumes (intravascular and total lung volume) is equal to the extravascular lung volume, which approximates to the extravascular lung water. The use of an ice-cold thermal bolus is thought to improve its ability to diffuse and thus make the measurement more accurate (Blindels et al 1999).

In acute lung injury, as in acute respiratory distress syndrome (ARDS), the hydrostatic pressure in the lungs alters, creating interstitial pulmonary edema. In any acute lung injury, this third spacing of fluid frequently occurs, decreasing the circulating volume. In this situation, the extravascular lung water would be expected to increase and intrathoracic blood volume to decrease (Lichtwarck-Ascoff et al 1992, Salukhe & Wyncoll 2002, Pitmann & Gupta 2003). The development of early pulmonary edema, with small changes in lung water, is often not detectable on a chest x-ray, or reflected in arterial blood gas analysis. This is because the chest x-ray is a two-dimensional representation of the density of the entire thorax, which makes the assessment of the amount of extravascular lung water present difficult to estimate clinically.

Cardiac function index

Assessment of the heart's ability to contract is important in the critically ill patient. Traditionally, this has been achieved using the pulmonary catheter by taking the ratio between the filling pressure (central venous or pulmonary artery) and the cardiac index, and the ejection fraction of the right ventricle. This is usually performed while giving a fluid challenge. The PiCCOplus provides an alternative to this method of assessing cardiac contractility by deriving the cardiac function index (CFI) from the ratio of the cardiac output to the global end-diastolic volume. The cardiac function index is independent of preload (Pittman & Gupta 2003).

Stroke volume variation and pulse pressure variation

The physiological explanation for the fluctuations in the arterial waveform, as a result of the interaction between the heart and lungs, have already been provided in detail in Chapter 5 (Pittman & Gupta 2003). The PiCCOplus displays the stroke volume variation (SVV) as a continuous parameter that has been derived from pulse contour analysis, as an indicator of fluid responsiveness to guide fluid therapy. However, it should be noted that the variation in stroke volume is only reliable in patients who are being ventilated mechanically with consistent tidal volumes.

Advantages and disadvantages of the PiCCOplus

When compared to the pulmonary artery catheter, the PiC-COplus is considered to be less invasive and, therefore, less of a risk to the patient. Most patients who are critically ill have central venous and arterial assess obtained as routine. Having said that, not all patients go on to require more in-depth cardiopulmonary monitoring and the PiCCOplus does require the insertion of its product-specific arterial line for this purpose (Pittman & Gupta 2003).

As with most cardiopulmonary hemodynamic monitors, there are some patient groups in which the use of a specific monitor is excluded. The use of the PiCCOplus is contra-indicated in patients who have restricted arterial access, either because of grafting of the femoral artery or those with severe burns to areas of choice for arterial access. Patients who have intracardiac shunts, aortic aneurysms or aortic stenosis, pneumonectomy or who are receiving extracorporeal membrane oxygenation therapy would generate inaccurate thermodilution measurements. The complications associated with the use of the PiCCOplus are related to those of cannulation of major arteries and veins.

In the event of significant alterations in the patient's heart rate, arterial blood pressure and vascular resistance, the pulse contour analysis has the potential to become unreliable. To overcome this, frequent recalibrations are necessary in order to allow for changes in aortic impedance.

REFERENCES

Afessa B, Spencer S, Khan W et al 2001 Association of pulmonary artery catheter use with in-hospital mortality. Critical Care Medicine 28: 1145–1148

Baele P L, McMichan J C, Marsh H M, Sil J C, Southorn P A 1982 Continuous mixed venous oxygen saturation in critically ill patients. Anesthesia Analogues 61: 513–517

Barash P G, Nardi D, Hammond G et al 1981 Catheter-induced pulmonary artery perforation: mechanisms, management, and modifications. Journal of Thoracic and Cardiovascular Surgery 82: 5–12

Barin E, Haryadi D G, Schokin S I et al 2000 Evaluation of a thoracic bioimpedance cardiac output monitor during cardiac catheterisation. Critical Care Medicine 28: 698–702

Bernard G R, Sopko G, Cerra F et al 2000 Pulmonary artery catheterization and clinical outcomes. National Heart, Lung and Blood Institute and Food and Drug Administration Workshop. JAMA 283: 2568–2572

Bindels A J G H, Van der Moeven J G, Meinders A E 1999 Pulmonary artery wedge pressure and extravascular lung water in patients with acute cardiogenic pulmonary oedema requiring mechanical ventilation. American Journal of Cardiology 85: 1158–1163

Birman H, Haq A, Hew E, Aberman A 1984 Continuous monitoring of mixed venous oxygen saturation in hemodynamically unstable patients. Chest 86: 753–756

Boldt J, Menges T, Wollbruck M et al 1994 Is continuous cardiac output measurement using thermodilution reliable in the critically ill patient? Critical Care Medicine 22: 1913–1918

Boyd K D, Thomas S J, Gold J, Boyd A D 1983 A prospective study of complications of pulmonary artery catheterizations in 500 consecutive patients. Chest 84: 245–249

Branthwaite M A, Bradley R D 1968 Measurement of cardiac output by thermal dilution in man. Journal of Applied Physiology 24: 434–438

Bridges E J 2000 Monitoring pulmonary pressures: just the facts. Critical Care Nurse 20(6): 59–78

Buchbinder N, Gunz W 1976 Hemodynamic monitoring: invasive techniques. Anesthesiology 45: 146–155

Buhre W, Weyland A, Buhre K et al 1993 Transoesophageal Doppler for continuous haemodynamic monitoring. British Journal of Intensive Care 3: 376–378

Cernaianu A C, Nelson L D 1993 The significance of mixed venous oxygen saturation and technical aspects of continuous measurement. In: Edwards J D, Shoemaker W C, Vincent J L (eds) Oxygen transport: principles and practice. WB Saunders, Philadelphia: 99–124

Connors A F, Speroff T, Dawson N V et al 1996 The effectiveness of right heart catheterization in the initial care of critically ill patients. JAMA 276: 889–897

Creed G M 2000 Can cardiac output be assessed clinically by intensive care staff? Care of the Critically Ill 16(3): 108–111

Critchley L A H 1998 Impedance cardiography. Anaesthesia 53: 677–684

Dalen J E, Bone R C 1996 Is it time to pull the pulmonary artery catheter? JAMA 276: 916–918

Darmon P-L, Hillel Z, Mogtader A, Mindich B, Thys D 1994 Cardiac output by transesophageal echocardiography using continuous wave Doppler across the aortic valve. Anesthesiology 80: 796–805

Darovic G O 2002 Hemodynamic monitoring: invasive and non invasive clinical applications, 3rd edn. Saunders, Philadelphia

DiCorte C J, Cathan P, Grelich P 2000 Esophageal Doppler monitor determination of cardiac output and preload during cardiac operations. Annals of Thoracic Surgery 69: 1782–1786

Dongre S S, McAslan T C, Shin B 1977 Selection of the source of mixed venous blood samples in severely traumatized patients. Anesthesia Analogues 56: 527–532

Edwards J D 1990 Practical application of oxygen transport principles. Critical Care Medicine 18: S45–S48

Edwards J D 1991 Oxygen transport in cardiogenic and septic shock. Critical Care Medicine 19: 658–663

Edwards J D, Mayall R M 1998 Importance of the sampling site for measurement of mixed venous oxygen saturation in shock. Critical Care Medicine 26: 1356–1360

Enger E L, Holm K 1990 Perspectives on the interpretation of continuous mixed venous oxygen saturation. Heart and Lung 19: 578–580

Fawcett J A D 2003 Nurse-led haemodynamic management: the patient's perspective. Care of the Critically Ill 19(2): 55–57

Garcia-Rodriguez C, Pittman J, Cassell C H, Sum-Ping J, El-Moalem H, Young C, Mark J B 2002 Lithium dilution cardiac output measurement: A clinical assessment of central venous and peripheral venous indicator injection. Critical Care Medicine 30: 2199–2204

Gawlinski A 1998 Can measurement of mixed venous oxygen saturation replace measurement of cardiac output in patients with advanced heart failure? American Journal of Critical Care 7(5): 374–380

Genoni M, Pelosi P, Romand J A, Pedoto A, Moccetti T, Malacrida R 1998 Determination of cardiac output during mechanical ventilation by electrical bioimpedance or thermodilution in patients with acute lung injury: effects of positive end-expiratory pressure. Critical Care Medicine 26: 1441–1445

Godje O, Hoke K, Goetz A E et al 2002 Reliability of a new algorithm for continuous cardiac output determination by pulse-contour analysis during hemodynamic instability. Critical Care Medicine 30: 52–58

Halfman S J, Noll M L 1990 Can continuous monitoring of mixed venous oxygen saturation be substituted for thermodilution cardiac output measurements? Focus on Critical Care 17: 157–158

Haller M, Zöllner C, Briegel J, Forst H 1995 Evaluation of a new continuous thermodilution cardiac output monitor in critically ill patients: a prospective criterion study. Critical Care Medicine 23: 860–866

Hassan E, Roffman D S, Applefeld M M 1987 The value of mixed venous oxygen saturation as a therapeutic indicator in the treatment of advanced CHF. American Heart Journal 113: 743–749

Hassan E, Green J A, Nara A R, Jarvis R C, Kasmer R J, Pospisil R 1989 Continuous monitoring of mixed venous oxygen saturation as an indicator of pharmacological intervention. Chest 95: 406–409

Headley J 1998 Invasive hemodynamic monitoring: applying advanced technologies. Critical Care Nursing Quarterly 21(3): 73–84

Hoeft A 1995 Transpulmonary indicator dilution: an alternative approach for hemodynamic monitoring. Yearbook of Intensive Care and Emergency Medicine, Springer-Verlag, Berlin: 593–605

Howard L, Gopinath S P, Uzura M, Valadka A, Robertson C S 1999 Evaluation of a new fiberoptic catheter for monitoring jugular venous oxygen saturation. Neurosurgery 44(6): 1280–1285

Imhoff M, Lehner H, Löhlein D 2000 Noninvasive whole-body electrical bioimpedance cardiac output and invasive thermodilution cardiac output in high-risk surgical patients. Critical Care Medicine 28: 2812–2818

Ivanov R, Allen J, Calvin J E 2000 The incidence of major morbidity in critically ill patient management with pulmonary artery catheters: a meta-analysis. Critical Care Medicine 28: 615–619

Jonas M 2001 Estimation of cardiac output. Critical care focus 6: cardiology in critical illness. British Medical Journal Books, London

Jonas M, Tanser S 2002a Estimation of changes in cardiac output from the arterial blood pressure waveform in the upper limb. British Journal of Anaesthesia 86, 4: 486–96

Jonas M, Tanser S 2002b Lithium dilution measurement of cardiac output and arterial pulse waveform analysis: an indicator dilution calibrated beat-by-beat system for continuous estimation of cardiac output. Current Opinion in Critical Care 8: 257–261

Jonas M M, Kelly F E, Linton R A F, Band D M, O'Brien T K, Linton N W F 1999 A comparison of lithium dilution cardiac output measurements made using central and antecubital venous injection of lithium chloride. Journal of Clinical Monitoring and Computing 15: 525–528

Jonas M, Hett D, Morgan J 2002 Real-time, continuous monitoring of cardiac output and oxygen delivery. International Journal of Intensive Care 9(Spring): 1

Kadota L 1986 Reproducibility of thermodilution cardiac output measurements. Heart and Lung 15: 618–622

Kouchoukos N T, Sheppard B S, McDonald D A 1970 Estimation of stroke volume in the dog by a pulse contour method. Circulation Research 26: 611–623

Kyff J V, Vaughn S, Yang S C, Raheja R, Puri V K 1989 Continuous monitoring of mixed venous oxygen saturation in patients with acute myocardial infarction. Chest 95: 607–611

Lake C L, Hines R L, Blitt C D 2001 Clinical monitoring: practical applications for anaesthesia and critical care. WB Saunders, Philadelphia

Leatherman J W, Shapiro R S 2003 Overestimation of pulmonary artery occlusion pressure in pulmonary hypertension due to partial occlusion. Critical Care Medicine 31: 93–97

Lefrant J Y, Bruelle P, Aya A G, Saïssi G, Dauzat M, de La Coussaye J E, Eledjam J J 1998 Training is required to improve the reliability of oesophageal Doppler to measure cardiac output in critically ill patients. Intensive Care Medicine 4: 347–352

Lichtwarck-Ascoff M, Zeravik J, Pfeiffer U J 1992 Intrathoracic blood volume accurately reflects circulatory volume status in critically ill patients with mechanical ventilation. Intensive Care Medicine 18: 142–147

Linton R A F, Band D M, Haire K M 1993 A new method of measuring cardiac output in man using lithium dilution. British Journal of Anaesthesia 71: 262–266

Linton R A F, Linton N W F, Band D M 1995 A new method of analysing indicator dilution curves. Cardiovascular Research 30: 930–938

Linton R A F, Band D M, O'Brien T K, Jonas M M, Leach R 1997 Lithium dilution cardiac output measurement: a comparison with thermodilution. Critical Care Medicine 25: 1796–1800

Linton R, Turtle M Band D, O'Brien T, Jonas M 1998 In vitro evaluation of a new lithium dilution method of measuring cardiac output and shunt fraction in patients undergoing venovenous extracorporeal membrane oxygenation. Critical Care Medicine 26: 174–177

Linton R A, Young L E, Marlin D J, Blissett K J, Brearley J C, Jonas Linton N W F, Linton R A F 2002 Haemodynamic response to a small intravenous bolus injection of epinephrine in cardiac surgical patients. European Journal of Anaesthesiology 19: 1–7

Marik P E, Pendelton J E, Smith R 1997 A comparison of hemodynamic parameters derived from transthoracic electrical bioimpedance with those parameters obtained by thermodilution and ventricular angiography. Critical Care Medicine 25: 1545–1550

Mark J B 1998 Atlas of cardiovascular monitoring. Churchill Livingstone. Edinburgh

Matthews P C, Nevin M 1998 Cardiac output measurement using the TECO1 oesophageal Doppler monitor. A comparison with thermodilution. International Journal of Intensive Care Autumn: 78–81

McKendry M, McGloin H, Saberi D, Caudwell L, Brady A R, Singer M 2004 Randomised controlled trial assessing the impact of a nurse delivered, flow monitored protocol for optimisation of circulatory status after cardiac surgery. British Medical Journal 329: 258

Nelson L D 1986 Continuous venous oximetry in surgical patients. Annals of Surgery 203: 329–333

Newman E V, Merrell M, Genecin A et al 1951 The dye dilution method for describing the central circulation. An analysis of factors shaping the time–concentration curves. Circulation 4: 735–746

Noll M L, Fountain R L 1990 The relationship between mixed venous oxygen saturation and cardiac output in mechanically ventilated coronary artery bypass graft patients. Progress in Cardiovascular Nursing 5: 34–40

Oates C 2001 Cardiovascular haemodynamics and Doppler waveforms explained. Greenwich Medical Media Ltd, London

O'Quin R, Marini JJ 1983 Pulmonary artery occlusion pressure: clinical physiology, measurement, and interpretation. American Review of Respiratory Disease 128: 319–326

Ott K, Johnson K, Ahrens T 2001 New technologies in the assessment of hemodynamic parameters. Journal of Cardiovascular Nursing 15(2): 41–55

Pearse R M, Ikram K, Barry J.G 2004 Equipment review: an appraisal of the LiDCO™plus method of measuring cardiac output. Critical Care 5 May.

Perrino A C, Harris S N, Luther M A 1998 Intraoperative determination of cardiac output using multiplane transesophageal echocardiography: a comparison to thermodilution. Anesthesiology 89: 350–357

Perruzzi W T, Gould R, Brodsky L 2001 Minimally invasive hemodynamic monitoring in: Vincent J L (ed) Yearbook of Intensive care and Emergency Medicine. Springer Heidelberg 2000, 481–490

Pfeiffer U J, Wisner-Euteneier A J, Lichtwarck-Ascoff M, Blumel G 1994 Less invasive monitoring of cardiac performance using arterial thermodilution. Clinical Intensive Care 5(Suppl): 28

Pinsky M R 2003a Pulmonary artery occlusion pressure. Intensive Care Medicine 29: 19–22

Pinsky M R 2003b Clinical significance of pulmonary artery occlusion pressure. Intensive Care Medicine 29: 175–178

Pittman J A L, Gupta K J 2003 Cardiac output monitoring: will new technologies replace the pulmonary artery catheter. In: Vincent J L (ed) Yearbook of Intensive Care and Emergency Medicine. Springer Heidelberg 481–490

Poelaert J, Schmidt C, Colardyn F 1998 Transoesophageal echocardiography in the critically ill. Anaesthesia 53: 55–68

Polanczyk C A, Rohde L E, Goldman L et al 2001 Right heart catheterization and cardiac complications in patients undergoing noncardiac surgery: an observational study. JAMA 286: 309–314

Pond C, Blessions G, Bowlin J, McCawley C, Lappas D 1992 Perioperative evaluation of a new mixed venous oxygen saturation catheter in cardiac surgical patients. Journal of Cardiovascular and Vascular Anesthesia 3: 280–282

Prentice D, Ahrens T 2001 Controversies in the use of the pulmonary artery catheter. Journal of Cardiovascular Nursing 15(2): 1–5

Rivers E, Nguyen B, Havstad S et al 2001 Early goal-directed therapy in the treatment of severe sepsis and septic shock. New England Journal of Medicine 345: 19: 1368–1377

Robin E D 1985 The cult of the Swan–Ganz catheter – use and abuse of pulmonary flow catheters. Annals of Internal Medicine 103: 445–449

Robin E D 1988 Defenders of the pulmonary artery catheter. Chest 93: 1059–1066

Rödig G, Prasser C, Keyl C, Liebold A, Hobbhahn J 1999 Continuous cardiac output measurement: pulse contour analysis vs thermodilution technique in cardiac surgical patients. British Journal of Anaesthesia 82: 525–530

Roizen M F, Berger D L, Gabel R A et al 1993 Practice guidelines for pulmonary artery catheterisation: a report by the American Society of Anesthesiologists task force on pulmonary artery catheterisation. Anesthesiology 8: 380–394

Sakka S G, Meier Hellmann A, Reinhart K 2000 Assessment of intrathoracic blood volume and extravascular lung water by single transpulmonary thermodilution. Intensive Care Medicine 26: 180–187

Salukhe T V, Wyncoll D L A 2002 Volumetric haemodynamic monitoring and continuous pulse contour analysis – an untapped resource for coronary and high dependency care units? British Journal of Cardiology (Acute and Interventional Cardiology) 9: 20–25

Sandham J, Hull R, Brant R et al 2003 A randomized, controlled trial of the use of pulmonary artery catheters in high risk surgical patients. New England Journal of Medicine 348: 5–14

Schmid E R, Spahn D R, Tornic M 1993 Reliability of a new generation transesophageal Doppler device for cardiac output monitoring. Anesthaesia Analogues 77: 971–979

Scuderi P E, MacGregor D A, Bowton D L, James R L 1994 A laboratory comparison of three pulmonary artery oximetry catheters. Anesthesiology 81: 245–253

Seeley R R 2000 Anatomy and physiology, 5th edn. WCB McGraw-Hill, California

Shoemaker W C, Velmahos G C, Demetriades D 2002 Procedures and monitoring for the critically ill. Saunders, Philadelphia

Silance P G, Simon C, Vincent J L 1994 The relation between cardiac index and oxygen extraction in acutely ill patients. Chest 105: 1190–1197

Sinclair S, James S, Singer M 1997 Intraoperative intravascular volume optimisation and length of hospital stay after repair of proximal femoral fracture: randomised controlled trial. British Medical Journal 315: 909–912

Singer M, Bennett E D 1991 Noninvasive optimization of left ventricular filling using esophageal Doppler. Critical Care Medicine 19: 1132–1137

Singer M, Allen M J, Webb A R, Bennett E D 1991 Effects of alterations in left ventricular filling, contractility and systemic vascular resistance on the ascending aortic blood velocity waveform of normal subjects. Critical Care Medicine 19: 1138–1145

Stetz C W, Miller R G, Kelly G E, Raffin T A 1982 Reliability of the thermodilution method in the determination of cardiac output in clinical practice. American Review of Respiratory Diseases 126: 1001–1004

Sturm J A 1990 Development and significance of lung water measurement in clinical and experimental practice. In: Lewis F R, Scuderi P E, MacGregor D A, Bowton D L, James R L. A 1994 Laboratory comparison of three pulmonary artery oximetry catheters. Anesthesiology 81: 245–253

Swan H J, Ganz W, Forrester J et al 1970 Catheterisation of the heart in man with use of a flow-directed balloon tipped catheter. New England Journal of Medicine 283: 447–451

Thomson G, Baker L, Mawby E, Leach R M 1996 Simultaneous comparison of five techniques of cardiac output measurement. Abstract in Intensive Care Medicine 22: S354

Treacher D F, Harvey C J, Bradley R D 1994 Can cardiac output be assessed clinically with sufficient accuracy to be of value in patient management? Comparison with thermodilution in intensive care unit patients. Abstract in Clinical Intensive Care 5: 12

Tuman K J, Carroll G C, Ivankovich A D 1989a Pitfalls in interpretation of pulmonary artery catheter data. Journal of Cardiothoracic Anesthaesiology 3: 625–641

Tuman K J, McCarthy R J, Speiss B D et al 1989b Effects of pulmonary artery catheterisation on outcome in patients undergoing coronary artery surgery. Anesthesiology 70:199–206

Valtier B, Cholley B P, Belot J P, de la Coussaye J E, Mateo J, Payen D M 1998 Noninvasive monitoring of cardiac output in critically ill patients using transesophageal Doppler. American Journal of Respiratory Critical Care Medicine 158: 77–83

Wesseling K H, Jansen J R, Settles J J, Schreuder J J 1993 Computation of aortic flow form pressure in humans using a nonlinear three-element model. Journal of Applied Physiology 74: 2566–2573

White K M 1991 Using continuous SVO_2 to assess oxygen supply/demand balance in the critically ill. Abbott Laboratories, North Chicago, IL

White K 2003 Fast Facts for adult critical care. Kathy White Learning Systems, Alabama

Wilson J, Woods I, Fawcett J et al 1999 Reducing the risk of major elective surgery: randomised controlled trial of preoperative optimisation of oxygen delivery. British Medical Journal 318: 1099–1103

Zollner C, Haller M, Weiss M et al 2000 Beat-to-beat measurement of cardiac output by intravascular pulse contour analysis: a prospective criterion standard study in patients after cardiac surgery. Journal of Cardiothoracic and Vascular Anesthesia 14: 125–129

FURTHER READING

Barone J E, Snyder A B 1991 Treatment strategies in shock: use of oxygen transport measurements. Heart and Lung 20: 81–85

Bazaral M G, Petre J, Novoa R 1992 Errors in thermodilution cardiac output measurements caused by rapid pulmonary artery temperature decreases after cardiopulmonary bypass. Anesthesiology 77: 31–37

Birch N J 1999 Inorganic pharmacology of lithium. Chemical Reviews 99: 2659–2682

Bland J M, Altman D G 1986 Statistical methods for assessing agreement between two methods of clinical measurement. Lancet February 8: 307–310

Boldt J, Heesen M, Muller M, Hemplemann G 1995 Continous monitoring of critically ill patients with a newly pulmonary arterial catheter. A cost analysis. Anaesthetist 44(6): 423–428

Calvin J E, Driedger A A, Sibbald W J 1981 Does the pulmonary capillary wedge pressure predict left ventricular preload in critically ill patients? Critical Care Medicine 9: 437–443

Cariou A, Monchi M, Dhainaut J F 1997 Continuous cardiac output and mixed venous saturation monitoring. Journal of Critical Care 13: 198–213

Copel L C, Stolarik 1991 A continuous SaO$_2$ monitoring: a research review. Dimensions of Critical Care Nursing 10: 202–209

Critchley L A H, Critchley J A J H 1999 A meta-analysis of studies using bias and precision statistics to compare cardiac output measurement techniques. Journal of Clinical Monitoring 15: 85–91

Dietzman R H, Ersek R A, Lillehei C W, Castaneda A R, Lillehei R C 1969 Low output syndrome: recognition and treatment. Journal of Thoracic Cardiovascular Surgery 57: 138–150

Dow P 1956 Estimations of cardiac output and central blood volume by dye dilution. Physiological Reviews 36: 77–102

Du Bois D, Du Bois E F 1916 A formula to estimate the approximate surface area if height and weight be known. Archives of Internal Medicine 17: 863–871

Eidelmann L A, Pizov R, Sprunh C L 1994 Pulmonary artery catheterization – at the crossroads? Critical Care Medicine 22: 543–545

Fegler G 1954 Measurement of cardiac output in anesthetized animals by a thermodilution method. Quarterly Journal of Experimental Physiology 39: 153–164

Field D 1997 Cardiovascular assessment. Nursing Times 93(35): 45–47

Fischer A P, Benis A M, Jurado R A, Seely E, Teirstein P, Litwak R S 1978 Analysis of errors in measurement of cardiac output by simultaneous dye and thermal dilution in cardiothoracic surgical patients. Cardiovascular Research 12: 190–199

Forrester J S, Ganz W, Diamond G, McHugh T, Chonette D W, Swan H J C 1972 Thermodilution cardiac output determination with a single flow-directed catheter. Americal Heart Journal 83: 306–311

Ganz W, Donoso R, Marcus H S, Forrester J S, Swan H J C 1971 A new technique for measurement of cardiac output by thermodilution in man. American Journal of Cardiology 27: 392–396

Godje O, Hoke K, Lichtwarck-Aschoff M, Lamm P, Reichart B 1999 Less invasive continuous cardiac output determination by femoral artery thermodilution calibrated pulse contour analysis: a comparison to conventional pulmonary arterial cardiac output. Critical Care Medicine 27(11): 2407–2412

Goldenheim P D, Kazemi H 1984 Cardiopulmonary monitoring of critically ill patients (parts 1 and 2). New England Journal of Medicine 311: 717–720, 776–780

Gomez C M H, Palazzo M G A 1998 Pulmonary artery catheterization in anaesthesia and intensive care. British Journal of Anaesthesia 81: 945–956

Gore J M, Goldberg R J, Spodick D H, Alpert J S, Dalen J E A 1987 Community-wide assessment of the use of pulmonary artery catheters in patients with acute myocardial infarction. Chest 92: 721–727

Gregory I C 1974 The oxygen and carbon monoxide capacities of foetal and adult blood. Journal of Physiology 236: 625

Gresham Bayne C 1997 Vital signs – are we monitoring the right parameter? Nursing Management 28(5): 74–76

Gunn S R, Pinsky M R 2001 Implications of arterial pressure variation in patients in the intensive care unit. Current Opinion in Critical Care 7: 212–217

Hamilton T T, Huber L M, Jessen M E 2002 PulseCO™: a less-invasive method to monitor cardiac output from arterial pressure after cardiac surgery. Annals of Thoracic Surgery 74: S1408–S1412

Hamilton W F, Remington J W 1947 The measurement of the stroke volume from the pressure pulse. American Journal of Physiology 148: 14–24

Hamilton W F, Moore J W, Kinsman J M, Spurling R G 1932 Studies on the circulation IV. Further analysis of the injection method, and of changes in hemodynamics under physiological and pathological conditions. American Journal of Physiology 99: 534–551

Headley J 1995 Strategies to optimize the cardiorespiratory status of the critically ill. AACN Clinical Issues 6(1): 121–134

Heerdt P M, Pond C G, Blessios G A, Rosenbloom M 1992 Inaccuracy of cardiac output by thermodilution during acute tricuspid regurgitation. Annals of Thoracic Surgery 53: 706–708

Hett D A, Jonas M M 2004 Non-invasive cardiac output monitoring. Intensive and Critical Care Nursing 20: 103–108

Horst H M, Obeid F N, Vij D, Bivins B A 1984 The risks of pulmonary artery catheterisation. Surgery, Gynecology and Obstetrics 159: 229–232

Imai T, Takahashi K, Fukura H, Morishita Y 1997 Measurement of cardiac output by pulse dye densitometry using indocyanine green: a comparison with the thermodilution method. Anesthesiology 84: 816–822

Ivanov R I, Allen J, Sandham J D, Calvin J E 1997 Pulmonary artery catheterisation: a narrative and systematic critique of randomised controlled trials and recommendations for the future. New Horizons 5: 268–276

Jakobsen C J, Melsen N C, Andresen E B 1995 Continuous cardiac output measurements in the perioperative period. Acta Anaesthesiologica Scandinavica 9: 485–488

Jonas M M, Kelly F E, Linton R A F, Band D M, O'Brien T K, Linton N W F 1999 A comparison of lithium dilution cardiac output measurements made using central and antecubital venous injection of lithium chloride. Journal of Clinical Monitoring and Computing 15: 525–528

Kelman G R 1966 Digital computer subroutine for the conversion of oxygen tension into saturation. Journal of Applied Physiology 21: 1375–1376

Kurita T, Morita K, Kawasaki H, Fujii K, Kazama T, Sato S 2002 Lithium dilution cardiac output measurement in oleic acid-induced pulmonary edema. Journal of Cardiothoracic and Vascular Anesthesia 16(3): 334–337

Linton R A F, Turtle M, Band D M, O'Brien T K, Jonas M M, Linton N W F 1999 A new technique for measuring cardiac output and shunt fraction during venovenous extracorporeal membrane oxygenation. Perfusion 14: 43–47

Lugo G, Arizpe D, Dominguez G, Ramirez M, Tamariz O 1993 Relationship between oxygen consumption and oxygen delivery during anesthesia in high-risk surgical patients. Critical Care Medicine 21:64–69

Mark J B 1995 Getting the most from your central venous pressure catheter. In: Barash PG (ed) ASA refresher courses in anaesthesiology, Vol. 23. Lippincott-Raven, Philadelphia: 157–175

Marx G T, Cope L, McCrossan S et al 2004 Assessing fluid responsiveness by stroke volume variation in mechanically ventilated patients with severe sepsis. European Journal of Anaesthesiology 21: 132–138

Model SAT-2 Oximeter/cardiac output operations manual [computer program]. Software version 7.12

Munro B H, Visintainer M A, Page E B 1986 Statistical methods for health care research. Philadelphia, JB Lippincott Co

Murdoch S D, Cohen A T, Bellamy M C 2000 Pulmonary artery catheterization and mortality in critically ill patients. British Journal of Anaesthesia 85: 611–615

Nightingale P 1990 Practical points in the application of oxygen transport principles. Intensive Care Medicine 16: S173–S177

Nishikawa T, Dohi S 1993 Errors in the measurement of cardiac output by thermodilution. Canadian Journal of Anaesthesia 40: 142–153

Parry-Jones A J D, Pittman J A L 2003 Arterial pressure and stroke volume variability as measurements for cardiovascular optimisation. International Journal of Intensive Care 10(2): 67–72

Pearson K S, Gomez M N, Moyers J R et al 1989 A cost/benefit analysis of randomised invasive monitoring for patients undergoing cardiac surgery. Anesthesia and Analgesia 69: 336–341

Polanczyk C A, Rohde L E, Goldman L et al 2001 Right heart catheterization and cardiac complications in patients undergoing noncardiac surgery: an observational study. JAMA 286: 309–314

Robin E D 1987 Death by pulmonary artery flow-directed catheter: time for a moratorium? (editorial) Chest 92: 727–731

Robin G D 1985 The cult of the Swan Ganz catheter. Overuse and abuse of pulmonary flow catheter. Anaesthetist International Medicine 103: 445–449

Sakka S G, Bredle D L, Reinhart K, Meier-Hellmann A 1999 Comparison of pulmonary artery and arterial thermodilution cardiac output in critically ill patients. Intensive Care Medicine 25: 843–846

Stamm R B, Carabello B A, Mayers D L et al 1982 Two dimensional echocardiographic measurement of left-ventricular ejection fraction: prospective analysis of what constitutes an adequate determination. American Heart Journal 104: 136–144

Stewart G N 1897 Researches on the circulation time and on the influences which affect it. Journal of Physiology 22: 159–183

Stow R W, Hetzel P S 1954 An empirical formula for indicator–dilution curves as obtained in human beings. Journal of Applied Physiology 7: 161–167

Sumimoto T, Takayama Y, Iwasaka T et al 1991 Mixed venous oxygen saturation as a guide to tissue oxygenation and prognosis in patients with acute myocardial infarction. American Heart Journal 122: 27–33

Sykes M K 1992 Clinical measurement and clinical practice. Anaesthesia 47: 425–432

Teboul J-L 2003 Dynamic concepts of volume responsiveness (Guest editorial). International Journal of Intensive Care Summer 10(2): 49–50

Thelan L A, Urden L D, Lough M E, Stacey K M 1998 Critical care nursing: diagnosis management, 3rd edn. Mosby, London

West J B, Dollery C T, Naimark A 1964 Distribution of blood flow in isolated lung: relation to vascular and alveolar pressures. Journal of Applied Physiology 19: 713

White H L 1947 Measurement of cardiac output by a continuously recording conductivity method. American Journal of Physiology 151: 45–57

White K M 1991 Using continuous SVO_2 to assess oxygen supply/demand balance in the critically ill. Abbott Laboratories, North Chicago, IL

Yelderman M L, Ramsay M A, Quinn M D, Paulsen A W, McKown R C, Gillman P H 1990 Continuous thermodilution cardiac output measurement in intensive care unit patients. Journal of Cardiothoracic and Vascular Anesthesia 6: 270–274

7 Optimization/ goal-directed therapy

Main objectives

- Highlight how each section in this book can be applied directly to patient care in order to improve outcome.
- Outline the background research that has led to current thinking on optimization/goal-directed therapy.
- Outline how nurses can take a lead role in the management of a patient's hemodynamic status using the evidence presented.

Introduction

Older patients with co-morbid disease, who undergo major surgical procedures, have significant morbidity and mortality, and represent a large proportion of patients requiring critical care in the UK (Campling et al 1992). In addition, survivors of high-risk surgery have been found to exhibit supranormal values of cardiac output, oxygen delivery and oxygen consumption when compared to non-survivors

(Shoemaker et al 1993). These facts have stimulated research activity in order to identify the 'at-risk' patient and evaluate a variety of interventions that aim to improve outcome.

'Optimization' and 'goal-directed therapy' are synonymous terms. The interest in this technique began back in the 1970s when Shoemaker and his colleagues demonstrated the link between achieving various cardiovascular end-points and the outcome of patients (Shoemaker, Montmomery & Kaplan et al 1973). In the UK, standard practice involves patients going straight to the operating theatre from their general ward, with the intraoperative monitoring being left to the judgement of the individual anesthetist managing the case, the nature of the surgery being undertaken and the potential for complications in the postoperative period. Major elective surgery has a significant impact on the occupancy of critical care and carries a significant mortality rate. The availability of beds in critical care is limited and can thus affect cancellation rates for surgery in high-risk cases (Wilson et al 1999).

Patients undergoing major elective surgery who have pre-existing limited cardiovascular reserve are more likely to have a poor outcome than those who do not (Boyd et al 1993). The improvements in anesthetic techniques over the last 40 years, in relation to staff, training, equipment, availability of monitoring and new drugs has influenced recovery (within the month following surgery), and outcome as a result of the anesthetic technique. It is now more likely for patients to die as a result of the surgery, rather than the anesthetic, and the individual patient's physiological reserve and, therefore, their ability to recover from it (Tuchschmidt et al 1992, Boyd et al 1993, Yu et al 1993).

During major surgery and the period afterwards, it is possible for both hypovolemia and hyoperfusion (common perioperatively) to be unrecognized. Generally, the effects become evident in the following days, as the body activates an inflammatory response to tissue hypoxia, affecting the normal functioning of major organs and tissues (Mythen & Webb 1995, Shoemaker et al 1999, Kern & Shoemaker 2002). In the presence of associated infection and endotoxemia, the normal inflammatory response augments and adds to the potential for multiorgan failure (McKendry et al 2004).

The cooperation that has developed between surgery and anesthesia has resulted in establishment of joint principles that favorably improve patient outcome, by minimizing complications resulting from tissue injury and by supporting tissue perfusion. Anesthetic techniques, historically, had not been standardized, and tended to rely on the preferences of individual anesthetists and be limited to all patients having similar surgery receiving the same routine management. Intraoperative monitoring, in general, was limited to the heart rate, blood pressure, central venous pressure and saturation of oxygen. These parameters provide no information about the adequacy of flow or tissue perfusion. However, it is anticipated that the increasing availability of hemodynamic technologies that enable the monitoring of flow during the perioperative period will favor outcome for patients generally (Singer & Bennett 1991, Sandman et al 2003).

History

Professor David Bennett at St George's Hospital, London, has been instrumental in the development of optimization practice and the dissemination of the findings from the many investigations and trials evaluating it as a means of improving outcome for patients after major surgery. The following section is based on the editorial written by

Bennett, which appeared in the *British Medical Journal* (1999), in which he gave a comprehensive review of the background and history of optimization.

Historically, cardiovascular physiology and the related control of the circulation is something taught early on, both in the medical and the nursing curriculum. Emphasis is put on the importance of arterial pressure, which provides very little information about flow. However, flow is important, in that it determines oxygen delivery (Boyd et al 1993).

The development of open-heart surgery in the 1950s demonstrated the importance of cardiac output for survival because it provided the opportunity to measure it. During the 1960s, the approach to optimizing flow focused on pharmacological and volume therapies, using right atrial pressure to assess filling and the temperature of the big toe to assess peripheral perfusion. The maximization of cardiac output continued to be advanced by the measurement of left atrial pressures and the use of dye dilution techniques. It was not long before both surgical and anesthetic teams applied these principles to the management of emergency and trauma patients (Newman, Merrell & Gerean 1951).

As the use of central venous pressure to assess and guide fluid therapy became accepted practice, the application to major elective surgical patients appeared to be a logical progression. However, the requirement for patients to be admitted to the critical care unit for the insertion of appropriate invasive lines, and the administration of fluid and drug therapies in order to prepare them, was not readily accepted. This was despite the publication of optimization studies demonstrating benefits to patients (Boyd et al 1993, Shoemaker, Appel & Kram 1993, Wilson et al 1999).

The concern about optimization and resistance to its acceptance in clinical practice revolved around the use of inotropes (following fluid loading), ordinarily used in emergency situations. Inotropes, such as adrenaline, are known to augment myocardial oxygen consumption, increasing the risk of myocardial ischemia. The change from inotropes to drive oxygen delivery to dilators, such as dopexamine, which may also reduce the inflammatory response, to assist oxygen delivery, followed (Wilson et al 1999). An additional issue was the concern about the use of the pulmonary artery catheter and the associated risks (Kuper and Soni 1996). To address this issue, some studies have utilized, and others are utilizing, alternative means of determining the adequacy of tissue perfusion (Rivers et al 2001, McKendry et al 2004). This seems to be the way forward (Bennett 1999).

The patient at risk

It is difficult to establish which patients are at 'high risk' absolutely. Having said that, there are two major determinants (the health of the patient and the nature of the surgery undertaken), established 'at-risk criteria' and several 'scoring systems' that attempt to do just that (Ball et al 2001). In addition, there is also the ability to estimate the physiological reserve of patients using cardiopulmonary exercise testing techniques prior to scheduling their surgery (Older et al 1993).

Older patients are at greater risk of increased mortality and morbidity (Campling et al 1992). This is because they have a higher number of concurrent disease processes and a decrease in their physiological reserve with aging (e.g. in their cardiac, renal, pulmonary and musculoskeletal systems). The type of surgery and its urgency can affect patient outcome considerably. It follows that patients who are sicker have higher mortality rates. Different procedures carry different mortality rates and emergency operations are known to have a higher mortality, particularly if a disease process is already underway prior to surgery. The difficulty is that not all patients fit into a category easily (Ball et al 2001, Vallet et al 2003).

Scoring systems

As a predictor of perioperative mortality, the American Society of Anesthesiologists physical status scale (ASA) is used widely. However, it does not put emphasis on the patient's cardiovascular status or differentiate between the dysfunctions of particular organs. In order to address the shortcomings of the ASA score, the Goldman index was developed (Goldman et al 1977). The Goldman index takes into consideration both risk of death and the prediction of a cardiac event.

The Acute Physiology and Chronic Health Evaluation score (APACHE; Knaus et al 1985) and the Physiological and Operative Severity Score for the enUmeration of Mortality and Morbidity (POSSUM; Copeland et al 1991) are also used. The APACHE score was not developed for the identification of the high-risk surgical patient. Having said that, in practice it is useful in the identification of patients who may need additional investigations in order to establish their fitness for surgery. The POSSUM score takes information about the patient's cardiac, respiratory and blood chemistry when assessing operative risk.

At-risk criteria

Several criteria for identifying patients at risk of high mortality and/or high morbidity have been developed. However, they all have emerged from the original criteria proposed by Shoemaker and his colleagues published in 1988. Since then, Shoemaker's criteria and variations on them have been used in several studies evaluating interventions to reduce both mortality and morbidity in surgical patients. These criteria can be subdivided into patient history, critical and surgical procedure factors (Vallet et al 2003). Shoemaker's criteria included patients over 70 years old with previous severe cardiorespiratory illness (acute myocardial infarction, chronic obstructive pulmonary disease, stroke, etc.) and patients undergoing extensive curative surgery for carcinoma (such as, esophagectomy, total gastrectomy), or surgery that lasted more than 8 hours.

Shoemaker also included patients who had severe multiple trauma (involving the opening of two body cavities or two organs) and those with significant acute blood loss. Finally, patients with shock, septicemia, acute renal or respiratory failure, those with late-stage vascular disease involving the aorta and any patients with an acute abdominal catastrophe resulting in their hemodynamic instability also fell into this category (Shoemaker et al 1993, Ball et al 2001).

It seems that, despite the availability and utilization of the numerous scoring systems, at-risk criteria and other more complex means of identifying 'at-risk' patients (some not covered in this book), a lack of agreement as to the most reliable method continues to exist (Ball et al 2001).

Aims of optimization/goal-directed therapy

The aim of optimization/goal-directed therapy is to reduce mortality, morbidity and the length of hospital care in those patients who are at risk of developing organ dysfunction, as a result of having undergone major, elective, emergency surgery and those with sepsis and septic shock, using different but specific end-points (Berlauk et al 1991, Boyd et al 1993, Wilson et al 1999). An additional aim of optimization/goal-directed therapy should be to achieve this with the least additional risk to the patient from the monitoring used, and the strategies employed. The problem is that, although numerous studies have evaluated optimization/goal-directed therapy, generally they have employed different strategies in different groups of patients, using different hemodynamic end-points; therefore, they have used different methods of estimating the adequacy of tissue perfusion.

The avoidance of the development of a tissue oxygen debt perioperatively, by using specific strategies (all of which include adequate fluid loading), has resulted in improvement in patient outcome (McKendry et al 2004). However, the use of some inotropes for this purpose, which are ordinarily reserved for emergency resuscitation (such as epinephrine), has come under criticism. This is because they are known to increase myocardial oxygen demand and may increase the likelihood of myocardial ischemia. The early hemodynamic assessment of a patient on the basis of physical findings, such as vital signs, central venous pressure and urinary output, fails to detect persistent global tissue hypoxia (Rivers et al 2001). During surgery, inadequate monitoring to allow for the evaluation of tissue oxygenation, excessive blood loss and falls in cardiac output is common. This increases the likelihood of complications developing (Wilson et al 1999).

Studies carried out in Canada and the USA, however, found no difference in postoperative outcome in patients with a pulmonary artery catheter and associated cardiac output monitoring. However, no specific end-points were targeted. This may reflect the difference between the UK and other countries where pulmonary artery catheters are routinely used and cardiac output monitored, particularly in cardiac surgery. These findings would seem to support the need to utilize monitoring appropriately (McKendry et al 2004), and be clear about what a clinician intends to achieve.

As already stated, optimization/goal-directed therapy has been used in patients with sepsis and septic shock within the critical care environment and in resuscitation/emergency rooms. This has involved achieving a balance between oxygen supply and demand, by manipulating preload, cardiac contractility and afterload (Shoemaker et al 1993, Berlauk et al 1991, Boyd et al 1993, Sinclair et al 1997, Wilson et al 1999). The rationale for instigating optimization/goal-directed therapy strategies in critically ill patients is to prevent the development of sepsis, which can lead to multiorgan failure, the development of long-term complications or death (Campling et al 1992, Gray et al 1997, Rivers et al 2001).

The systemic inflammatory response is a normal homeostatic mechanism triggered by the need to protect the body from some insult. In general, this is self-limiting. However, in certain situations, it can progress to the development of sepsis and septic shock (Rivers et al 2001). Global tissue hypoxia or shock is an important occurrence in the development of multiorgan failure and death. It results from an imbalance between the delivery of oxygen and the tissue demand or need for it. An imbalance can be attributed to several causes, such as hypovolemia (intravascular fluid depletion), myocardial depression, peripheral vasodilation and a rise in the metabolic rate. In addition to stimulating the inflammatory response, global tissue hypoxia also contributes to the activation of the endothelium. This interferes with the key mechanisms leading to failure of the microcirculation, refractory tissue hypoxia and organ dysfunction, such as the homeostatic balance in coagulation, and the permeability and tone of the vasculature (Rivers et al 2001).

The time frame for the move to severe critical illness is often referred to as the 'golden hours' (Rivers et al 2001). These may pass by while the patient is on a ward, in the resuscitation/emergency room, or in the critical care unit, if its development goes unrecognized, and treatment options that could have influenced outcome favorably may be futile (Rivers et al 2001).

The emphasis here is on early recognition and early initiation of appropriate treatments. In the case of the high-risk surgical patient, preoperative 'work-up' or optimization/goal-directed therapy may maximize tissue perfusion before a surgical insult. Further intraoperative and postoperative monitoring and management of tissue perfusion using appropriate techniques should follow. The ultimate strategy in achieving the balance between oxygen supply and demand is the use of goal-orientated proactive manipulation of the components of cardiac output (preload, contractility and afterload), and appropriate end-points to confirm that this balance has been achieved. The monitoring systems used to obtain these data (see Chapter 6) will depend on preferences and availability of equipment in individual departments. These end-points may include the achievement of normal values for cardiac output and oxygen delivery, and the analysis of arterial blood for lactate concentrations, base deficit and the pH. In addition, mixed venous oxygen saturation, as a surrogate for cardiac index, can be used as an appropriate end-point. As stated previously, venous oxygen saturation can be obtained from the central circulation, if the insertion of a pulmonary artery catheter is impractical or undesirable (McKendry et al 2004).

The incidence of septic shock has increased gradually over the past few decades. However, mortality rates associated with septic shock have changed little (decreased slightly). Studies that have been conducted using hemodynamic parameters as end-points, with negative results, have prompted the suggestion that future research should focus on patients who have global hypoxia as a result of similar causes and that this should be conducted at an earlier stage in the disease process (Rivers et al 2001). In terms of outcome, the benefits of optimization/goal-directed therapy can be attributed to a multitude of factors. Patients who received standard therapy, in the study conducted by Rivers and his colleagues (2001), had double the incidence of death (owing to sudden cardiovascular collapse) than those who benefited from 'early' goal-directed therapy. From these results, it was concluded that the move from severe disease can be rapid, and an important cause of early death (Rivers et al 2001).

If patients who have stable vital signs, and yet have already developed global tissue hypoxia, are identified and treated early, the subsequent need for invasive and supportive therapy (with the associated risks) may be avoided (Rivers et al 2001). On an economic note, this will obviously impact positively on costs and may balance out with the cost of optimization/early goal-directed therapy provided earlier.

Nurse-led hemodynamic monitoring

There is a great deal of evidence to support the early initiation of optimization/goal-directed therapy in order to restore and maintain the balance between the supply of oxygen to the tissues and the tissues demand for oxygen. This impacts on patient outcome by reducing mortality and morbidity, and length of hospital stay, and has become the cornerstone of the management of both the critically ill and the major elective surgical patient (Boyd, Grounds & Bennett 1993, Wilson et al 1999, McKendry et al 2004).

The hemodynamic management of patients is increasingly being nurse led. The last few years have seen the emergence of technologies that guide fluid therapy, including utilizing heart–lung interactions during mechanical ventilation (Pinsky 2003b) and Doppler waveforms (McKendry et al 2004). When compared to central venous and pulmonary artery occlusion pressure, these have been found to be more reliable monitors and predictors of hypovolemia (Pinsky 2003b). In order to manage the hemodynamic status of these patients using these new techniques, nurses need to understand the theoretical principles behind them.

Practicalities

It is important to define what is meant by 'nurse led'. Decisions about treatment regimes, and the monitors utilized to generate the appropriate data to decide on them, will ultimately lie with the clinician responsible for the patient. Having said that, hemodynamic monitors that can be initiated, set up, calibrated and totally managed by the nurse at the bedside can be defined as being nurse led. The addition of appropriate and specific protocols and/or guidelines for fluid and vasoconstrictor/dilator administration and titration by nurses enhances this.

It makes sense for the hemodynamic management of patients to be nurse led. Nurses are at the bedside most of the time, and are familiar with the hemodynamic monitoring technology available for use and the calibration procedures that they rely upon for accuracy. Nurse education for critical care nurses is widely available and includes in-depth coverage of cardiorespiratory physiology, pharmacology and pathophysiology. In addition, many critical care nurses have a great deal of critical care experience and are used to the potential effects of drugs used in the critically ill. However, not all critical care nurses have the benefit of this education and experience, and this needs to be taken into account when deciding on the use of protocols, which should be followed without deviation, and guidelines, which allow for a certain amount of clinical judgement.

Pulmonary artery catheter

The nurse's experience of trying to manage the fluid status of patients, by targeting a pressure end-point (pulmonary capillary wedge pressure; PCWP) that required right heart catheterization, presented its own problems. Firstly, timing was often affected by the availability of a doctor to put the pulmonary artery catheter in, so that the nurse could begin the hemodynamic management. Secondly, the PCWP proved to be a poor predictor and monitor of patient's fluid status clinically (Fawcett 2003). Some patients were given large volumes of fluid to try to increase and maintain the PCWP according to the protocol being used. However, in many cases, patients simply increased their urine output until the fluid load was lost from the systemic circulation, making it impossible to achieve PCWP targets (Fawcett 2004).

This made the use of a prescribed fluid and inotrope protocol unsafe without the nurse exercising sound clinical judgement. This led to an interest in more reliable, less invasive methods of achieving the same end-points (Fawcett 2004).

In contrast, the LiDCOplus™ (Lithium InDicator Cardiac Output Plus) for continuous pulse power analysis in association with a lithium calibration as an alternative to the pulmonary artery catheter can be completely managed by nurses, regardless of experience. It has been found to be quick and easy to set up and to calibrate (with some practice). Hemodynamic data are then available with minimal delay because it does not require a doctor (who may be busy elsewhere) to be involved in the process. However, as previously stated, decisions about treatment regimes (using protocols or guidelines) based on this and on any other monitored data still lie with the individual clinician responsible for the patient.

Patients who had undergone active preoptimization using the pulmonary artery catheter were surveyed (96 replies out of 138). Many of the patients found the process unpleasant, particularly the insertion of the pulmonary artery catheter and, for some patients, administration of large amounts of intravenous fluids prior to surgery. The achievement of supranormal flow (cardiac output) values was made, however, and resulted in improved outcome for these patients (Fawcett 2003). Despite their appreciation of the one to one nursing they received preoperatively, in the critical care unit, there were many additional practical problems for patients (e.g. bowel preparation and the environment, including noise). Most patients stated that they had not realized what it was going to be like and would not like to repeat the experience again (Fawcett 2003).

Using Doppler

McKendry and her colleagues (2004) reported the use of a nurse-led protocol in order to optimize the circulatory status of patients who were in the early stages of recovery from cardiac surgery. The protocol involved the use of esophageal Doppler flowmetry, with the probe being inserted and positioned correctly by nurses (see Chapter 6) without assistance from clinicians. Stroke volume was targeted and improved using the size of the waveform as a guide. The protocol was associated with a trend towards a reduced length of hospital stay and fewer complications, and suggested that a nurse-led, protocol-driven approach could have widespread application (McKendry et al 2004).

Summary

As already stated, the hemodynamic management of critically ill patients is increasingly being nurse led. At the same time, the way the hemodynamic status of patients is managed is changing, with various means of measuring and monitoring flow that are less invasive increasingly being used. The estimation of left ventricular performance is still an important aspect in the diagnosis and management of the critically ill (Pinsky 2003b), but the way it is measured or estimated is changing.

There is strong evidence suggesting that the hemodynamic management of patients using pressure end-points is less effective than flow. Heart–lung interactions as a reliable means of identifying those who need fluid and the effects of a fluid load on stroke volume are an attractive option. However, nurses need to understand the underlying physiology of the cardiovascular system and how it is affected by mechanical ventilation, if they are to utilize alternative technologies to achieve this. An appreciation of the limitations of these heart–lung interactions is essential.

The ability to recognize when homeostatic mechanisms have been triggered in a critically ill patient is important. When

> ## Quiz 7.1
>
> 1. *Do you know what optimization/goal-directed therapy is?*
> 2. *What does it aim to achieve?*
> 3. *How can it be nurse led?*
> 4. *How would you go about doing that in your own unit?*

evaluating hemodynamic monitored data, it has to be remembered that adequate pressure does not necessarily reflect adequacy of flow. Similarly, adequate flow does not ensure the delivery of oxygen to the tissues or influence the ability of the cells to utilize the oxygen it is receiving. This has led to a great deal of research being done on monitoring the microcirculation and, in particular, the role of the mitochondria.

Implementing nurse-led hemodynamic management should be a multidisciplinary decision, including the involvement of nurses in the decision-making about the type of monitors being considered for use. A clear agreement should be made about what is and what is not required, expected or desirable for nurses to do. Implementation of any new practice, monitoring equipment or protocol/guideline can be problematic and the identification of key individual nurses for support can be extremely helpful. Finally, most manufacturers of hemodynamic monitors provide or guide users of their equipment to appropriate support, education and training (via the monitor itself or in materials) and advantage should be taken of these.

Summary

There is substantial evidence to support the improvement in postoperative outcome by the maintenance of adequate tissue perfusion. Unfortunately, implementing this in practice places additional pressure on critical care facilities and beds. In comparison to the rest of a hospital, critical care tends to have more staff. The ratio of patient to nurse varies from hospital to hospital, and country to country, but is often one to one.

Critical care is limited in its availability to all patients. This is because of cost and resource limitations. Because of this, it seems logical to concentrate what resources are available on those patients who will benefit, in terms of outcome, from its treatment options (Bennett 1999). The development of services and monitoring equipment available outside the walls of specialized critical care units may take some of the pressure off these units, by enabling the earlier recognition and instigation of treatments, thus avoiding admission to the critical care environment itself. Although some contradictions do exist, the body of knowledge supporting the active optimization of patients using a variety of interventions is increasing and demonstrating substantial positive impact on patient outcome (Bennett 1999). Unfortunately, there are obstacles to changing practice and recognizing the benefits of providing critical care facilities for patients following high-risk surgery despite the evidence to support it (Berlauk et al 1991, Boyd et al 1993, Bishop et al 1995, Wilson et al 1999, Takala et al 2000). Often the problem arises from the accident and emergency departments having difficulty finding critical care beds, necessitating the cancellation of major elective surgery, or the even more worrying situation of operating and then sending patients back to general surgical wards (Bennett 1999).

Optimization (goal-directed therapy) has also shown benefits for patients in the early stages of severe sepsis and septic shock, although, when compared to overall hospital stay for patients, the benefits in both the short and long term are significant. The emphasis here is on 'early' identification of those patients who are at high risk of an imbalance between oxygen supply and demand, and from overall cardiovascular collapse, with the timing and quality of resuscitation being an important consideration for future research (Rivers et al 2001).

REFERENCES

Ball J, Rhodes A, Bennett E D 2001 Reducing the morbidity and mortality of high-risk surgical patients. In: Vincent J L (ed.) Yearbook of intensive care and emergency medicine, Springer, Heidelberg: 331–342

Bennett E D 1999 Editorial, British Medical Journal, Medical Journal 318

Berlauk J F, Abrams J H, Gilmour I J, O'Connor S R, Knighton D R, Cerra F B 1991 Preoperative optimization of cardiovascular hemodynamics improves outcome after peripheral vascular surgery. A prospective, randomised clinical trial. Annals of Surgery 214: 289–297

Bishop M H, Shoemaker W A, Appel P L 1995 Prospective, randomised trial of survivor values of cardiac index, oxygen delivery and oxygen consumption as resuscitation endpoints in severe trauma. Journal of Trauma 38: 780–787

Boyd O, Grounds M, Bennett E D 1993 A randomized clinical trial of the effect of deliberate perioperative increase of oxygen delivery on mortality in high-risk surgical patients. JAMA 270: 2699–2707

Campling E A, Delvin H B, Hoile R W, Lunn J N 1992 Enquiry into peri-operative deaths. Royal College of Surgeons, London

Copeland G P, Jones M W 1991 POSSUM: a scoring system for surgical audit. British Journal of Surgery 78: 355–360

Fawcett J A D 2004 Haemodynamic monitoring: heart-lung interactions. Care of the Critically Ill 20(2): 38–41

Fawcett J A D 2003 Nurse-led haemodynamic management: the patient's perspective. Care of the Critically Ill 19(2): 55–57

Goldman L, Caldera D L, Nussbaum S R 1977 Multifactoral index of cardiac risk in noncardiac surgical procedures. New England Journal of Medicine 297: 845–850

Gray A J, Hoile R W, Ingram G S, Sherry K M 1997 The report of the National Confidential Enquiry into Perioperative Deaths 1996/1997. Royal College of Surgeons, London: 118

Kern J W, Shoemaker W C 2002 Meta analysis of hemodynamic optimisation in high risk patients. Critical Care Medicine 30: 1686–1699

Knaus W A, Draper E A, Wagner D P et al 1985 APACHE II: a severity of disease classification system. Critical Care Medicine 13: 818–829

Kuper M, Soni N 2003 Equipment review: Non invasive Cardiac Output Monitors CPD in Anaesthesia 5:1: 17–25

McKendry M, McGloin H, Saberi D, Caudwell L, Brady A R, Singer M 2004 Randomised controlled trial assessing the impact of a nurse delivered, flow monitored protocol for optimisation of circulatory status after cardiac surgery. British Medical Journal 329: 433–438

Mythen M G, Webb A R 1995 Peroperative plasma volume expansion reduces the incidence of gut mucosal hypoperfusion in cardiac surgery. Archives of Surgery 130: 423–429

Newman E V, Merrel M, Genecin A et al 1951 The dye dilution method for describing the central circulation: An analysis of factors shaping the time-concentration curves. Circulation 4: 735–746

Older P, Smith R, Courtney P, Hone R 1993 Preoperative evaluation of cardiac failure and ischemia in elderly patients by cardiopulmonary exercise testing. Chest 104: 701–704

Pinsky M R 2003a Pulmonary artery occlusion pressure. Intensive Care Medicine 29: 19–22

Pinsky M R 2003b Clinical significance of pulmonary artery occlusion pressure. Intensive Care Medicine 29: 175–178

Rivers R, Nguyen B, Havstad S et al 2001 Early goal-directed therapy in the treatment of severe sepsis and septic shock. New England Journal of Medicine 345, 19: 1368–1377

Sandham J D, Hull R D, Brant R F et al 2003 A randomised, controlled trial of the use of pulmonary artery catheters in high risk surgical patients. New England Journal of Medicine 348: 5–14

Shoemaker W C, Montgomery E S, Kaplan E, Elwyn D H 1973 Physiologic patterns in surviving and non surviving shock patients. Use of sequential cardiorespiratory variables in defining criteria for therapeutic goals and early warning of death. Archives of Surgery 106: 630–636

Shoemaker W C, Apple P L, Kram H B 1993 Hemodynamic and oxygen transport responses in survivors and non-survivors of high risk surgery. Critical Care Medicine 21: 977–990

Shoemaker WC, Thangathurai D, Velmahos G et al 1999 Haemo-dynamic patterns of survivors and non survivors during high risk elective surgical operations. World Journal of Surgery 23: 1264–1270

Sinclair S, James S, Singer M 1997 Intraoperative intravascular volume optimisation and length of hospital stay after repair of proximal femoral fracture: randomised controlled trial. British Medical Journal 315: 909–912

Singer M, Bennett E D 1991 Noninvasive optimization of left ven-tricular filling using esophageal Doppler. Critical Care Medicine 19: 1132–1137

Takala J, Meier-Hellman A, Eddelston J, Hulstaert P, Sramek V 2000 Effect of dopexamine on outcome after major abdominal surgery: a prospective randomised, controlled multicentre study. European Multicentre Study Group on Dopexamine in major elec-tive abdominal surgery, Critical Care Medicine 28: 3417–3423

Tuchschmidt J, Fried J, Astiz M, Rackow E 1992 Elevation of cardiac output and oxygen delivery improves outcome in septic shock. Chest 102: 216–220

Vallet B, Lebuffe G, Weil E 2003 High-risk surgical patients: why we should pre-optimise? In: Vincent J L (ed.) Yearbook of inten-sive care and emergency medicine. Springer, Heidelberg 331–342

Wilson J, Woods I, Fawcett J et al 1999 Reducing the risk of major elective surgery: randomised controlled trial of preoperative opti-misation of oxygen delivery. British Medical Journal 318: 1099–1103

Yu M, Levy M M, Smith P, Takiguchi S A, Miyasaki A, Myers S A 1993 Effect of maximizing oxygen delivery on morbidity and mor-tality rates in critically ill patients: a prospective, randomized, con-trolled study. Critical Care Medicine 21: 830–838

SUGGESTED READING

Berne R M, Levy M N 2001 Cardiovascular physiology, 8th edn. Mosby, London

Criner G J, Alonzo E D 1999 Pulmonary pathophysiology. Black-well Science Inc, Oxford

Gawlinski A 1998 Can measurement of mixed venous oxygen satura-tion replace measurement of cardiac output in patients with advanced heart failure? American Journal of Critical Care 7: 374–380

Gunn S R, Pinsky M R 2001 Implications of arterial pressure vari-ation in patients in the intensive care unit. Current Opinion in Critical Care 7: 212–217

Harrigan P, Pinsky M 2001 Heart-lung interactions. Part 2: effects of intra-thoracic pressure. International Journal of Intensive Care 8: 99–108

Hayes M A, Timmins A C, Yau E H S, Palazzo M, Hinds C J, Watson D 1994 Elevation of systemic oxygen delivery in the treatment of critically ill patients. New England Journal of Medicine 330: 1717–1722

Kusumoto F M 1999 Cardiovascular pathophysiology. Blackwell Science Inc, Oxford

Lake C L, Hines R L, Blitt C D 2001 Clinical monitoring: practical applications for anaesthesia and critical care. Saunders, Philadelphia

Michard F, Teboul J L 2000 Using heart–lung interactions to assess fluid responsiveness during mechanical ventilation. Critical Care 4: 282–289

Michard F, Teboul J L 2002 Predicting fluid responsiveness in ICU patients: a critical analysis of the evidence. Chest 121: 2000–2008

Mythen M G, Webb A R 1995 Perioperative plasma volume expansion reduces the incidence of gut mucosal hypoperfusion during cardiac surgery. Archives of Surgery 130: 423–429

Oates C 2001 Cardiovascular haemodynamics and Doppler waveforms explained. Greenwich Medical Media Ltd, London

Parry-Jones A J D, Pittman J A L 2003 Arterial pressure and stroke volume variability as measurements for cardiovascular optimisation. International Journal of Intensive Care Summer 10(2): 67–72

Rook G A, Schwid H A, Shapira Y 1995 The effect of graded haemorrhage and intravascular volume replacement on systolic pressure variation in humans during mechanical and spontaneous ventilation. Anaesthesia and Analgesia 80: 925–932

Tavernier B, Makhotine O, Lebuffe G 1998 Systolic pressure variation as a guide to fluid therapy in patients with sepsis-induced hypotension. Anaesthesiology 89: 1313–1321

White K 2003 Fast Facts for adult critical care,. Kathy White Learning Systems, Alabama

Wiesenack C, Prasser C, Rodig G, Kely C 2003 Stroke volume variation as an indicator of fluid responsiveness using pulse contour analysis in mechanically ventilated patients. Cardiovascular Anaesthesia 96: 1254–1257

Woods S L, Froelicher E S S, Adams S 2000 Cardiac nursing, 4th edn. Lippincott, Philadelphia

Clinical scenario 3

Harriet Sommes is a 35-year-old lady who has a previous medical history of considerable alcohol and drug abuse. She was admitted to the critical care unit in the early hours of the morning with sepsis secondary to a severe chest infection. She is currently on non-invasive ventilation via a simple CPAP circuit with 5 cmH$_2$O.

You have just arrived for the day shift. You had been told at handover that she had been tachycardic at a rate of 135 with an arterial blood pressure of 90/56 for much of the time since admission. She is drowsy but complaining of thirst. Her temperature is 39.1°C. Despite a total of 1500 ml in fluid (colloid and crystalloid) over the last 2 hours, she remains tachycardic and her blood pressure is now 88/44 (arterial line in situ). This has just occurred according to the nurse handing over. Harriet only has one peripheral line.

- Have this lady's homeostatic mechanisms been triggered?
- How do you know?
- How would you assess the accuracy of all the monitoring systems in use in this scenario?
- How might you optimize the data generated by the monitoring systems in use?
- What further information would help you to assess her central and peripheral perfusion?
- What additional technology could you use in this situation, and how would it benefit Harriet?
- How would you approach management of her hemodynamic status within the constraints of the organization you work in now?
- Given the freedom to change these constraints, how would you manage her hemodynamic status in order to improve her mortality, morbidity and length of hospital stay, while maintaining Harriet's individual needs?

For answers, see Appendix 2 (page 233).

APPENDICES

APPENDIX I
Knowledge reviews

SECTION 1

1. Do you know the location, size and position of the heart in the thoracic cavity?
2. Are you able to identify the layers of the heart and describe their function?
3. Can you identify the heart chambers, sounds and valves, and discuss the functions of each?
4. Can you trace blood flow through the heart and compare the functions of the heart chambers on the right and left sides?
5. Are you able to discuss the blood supply to the heart?
6. Can you describe the effects of the autonomic nervous system on heart function?
7. Can you list the anatomical components of the heart's conduction system?
8. Are you able to identify the electrical events associated with the normal electrocardiogram?
9. Can you explain the mechanical events of the cardiac cycle?

SECTION 2

1. Can you state what cardiac output is and describe the factors that affect it?
2. Are you able to explain how cardiac output is controlled and regulated?
3. Can you explain the meaning of the terms preload, afterload and contractility?
4. Can you distinguish between the structure and function of arteries, veins and capillaries?

5. Are you able to explain the mechanisms involved in the regulation of blood flow?

6. Can you describe how blood pressure is controlled and regulated?

7. Can you discuss the pressures involved in the movement of fluids across compartments?

SECTION 3

1. Can you identify the principles of biological sensors and monitoring?

2. Are you able to outline the indications for continuous monitoring?

3. Can you recognize the indications for arterial cannulation, insertion sites and complications?

4. Are you able to recognize the limitations of monitoring systems?

5. Can you provide an outline of the indications for central venous cannulation?

6. Do you recognize the limitations of central venous pressure measurement?

7. Are you able to recognize the information that can be obtained from the pulmonary artery catheter?

8. Do you feel you now have a working knowledge of arterial and CVP waveform morphology?

9. Are you able to outline the principles underpinning a range of hemodynamic monitors?

10. Can you identify the parameters each monitor measures?

11. Can you list the advantages and disadvantages of each monitoring system?

12. Are you able to identify the potential uses of each monitor in different clinical situations?

13. Do you know what optimization/goal-directed therapy is?

14. Do you understand the reasons for optimization/goal-directed therapy?

15. Can you see how it can be successfully nurse led and how to go about doing it?

APPENDIX 2
Answers to clinical scenarios

Recognizing when homeostatic mechanisms have been triggered is important.

The nurse is the best monitor
Look:
- capillary refill
- conscious level
- urine output.

Listen:
- patient.

Feel:
- pulse
- skin temperature.

ECG monitoring
The ECG only shows electrical activity:
- dysrhythmias
- ischemia
- electrolyte imbalances
- drug toxicity.

It does not show:
- cardiac output
- tissue perfusion.

Non-invasive blood pressure
- Tends to overestimate at low pressure/underestimate at high pressure/give erroneous results in atrial fibrillation or with other arrhythmias.

- Cuff width is an important determinant of the accuracy (should be 40% of mid-circumference of limb and the length should be twice the width).
- Too narrow a cuff overestimates and too wide a cuff underestimates pressure.

Urine output

- Strictly speaking, this is a monitor of renal perfusion only: urine output is often used as a guide to adequacy of cardiac output as the kidney receives 25% of cardiac output.
- When renal perfusion is adequate, urine output will exceed 0.5 ml/kg per hour.
- Use of diuretics, such as frusemide and dopamine, abolishes its usefulness as a hemodynamic monitor.

Hemodynamic waveform interpretation

- This is most accurately measured on a graphic recorder using two-channel paper recorder to record ECG simultaneously with waveforms to improve identification of waveform characteristics.
- The paper should have at least 2 inches per channel printout of scale to allow precise measurement of the pressure value.
- Measure waveforms at end-expiration.
- Locate end-expiration:
  - For spontaneous breathing, locate the waveform just before pressures decline with inhalation.
  - For mechanical breathing, locate the waveform just before the pressure rise with inhalation.
- For the electronic fluid-filled system to measure pressures accurately, the pressure signal from the patient must be transmitted through an unobstructed fluid system, and the transducer must be zeroed, levelled and calibrated if necessary.
- The frequency response and damping characteristics of the system must also be optimized.

Arterial waveform: relationship to ECG
- Delays (120–180 ms);
- spread of electrical depolarization through the ventricle;
- isovolumetric contraction;
- aortic valve opening;
- left ventricular ejection;
- transmission of the aortic pressure wave to the radial artery;
- transmission of the pressure signal from the arterial line to the pressure transducer.

Site of arterial line
- Pressure waves recorded simultaneously from different sites have different morphologies.
- As the arterial blood pressure travels from the central aorta to the periphery several characteristic changes occur:
  - the arterial upstroke is steeper
  - the systolic peak is higher
  - dicrotic notch appears later
  - the diastolic wave is more prominent
  - the end-diastolic pressure is lower
  - the mean arterial pressure is accurately monitored.

Ventilated patients
Rises and falls in hemodynamic pressure waveform components are related to mechanical activities of the heart and are caused by:
- changes in blood volume (blood entering or exiting a chamber or a vessel);
- changes in myocardial tension – muscle fibers are contracting (systole) or relaxing (diastole);
- changes in intrathoracic pressure (mechanical events are preceded by corresponding electrical events – they correlate with the ECG).

Systolic pressure variation

- In mechanically ventilated patients, the effect of positive intrathoracic pressure during inspiration is to increase left ventricular output and systolic arterial pressure early in inspiration, followed a few heartbeats later by a fall.
- This variation in arterial pressure is exaggerated in the presence of reduced preload, and a significant correlation has been demonstrated between the systolic arterial pressure variations and the end-diastolic area estimated with transesophageal echocardiography.
- It can be quantified by establishing a baseline during a period of apnea and then measuring the maximum subsequent upward (d up) and downward (d down) variation.
- It provides better prediction of the responsiveness to fluid loading than pulmonary capillary wedge pressure and left ventricular end-diastolic area owing to a transient fall in venous return.
- It occurs in early inspiration owing to the augmentation of stroke volume because of the increase in left-sided preload.
- In patients with impaired left ventricular contractility, it may also reflect the afterload reducing effect of positive intrathoracic pressure.

Pulse pressure variation

- This is defined as the maximal pulse pressure less the minimum pulse pressure divided by the average of these two pressures.
- It is thought to reflect changes more accurately in left ventricular stroke work because it is not influenced by the intrathoracic pressure-induced changes in the arterial pulse.

APPENDIX 3
Equations

I. THE THERMODILUTION CARDIAC OUTPUT EQUATION

$$Q = \frac{V(TB - TI)K1K2}{TB(d)dt}$$

where Q is cardiac output, V is volume injected, TB is blood temperature, TI is injectate temperature, K1 and K2 are computational constants, and TB(t)dt is the change in blood temperature as a function of time.

2. THE FICK EQUATION

$$\text{Cardiac output} = \frac{\text{Oxygen consumption}}{\text{Arteriovenous oxygen difference}}$$

or

$$CO = \frac{VO_2}{ADVO_2}$$

APPENDIX 4
Cardiac calculations

1. $SV = (CO/HR) \times 1000$ (ml)

where SV is the stroke volume, CO is the cardiac output (liters/min) and HR is the heart rate (beats/min).

2. $SVI = (CI/HR) \times 1000$ (ml/m²)

where SVI is the stroke volume index, CI is the cardiac index (liters/min per m²) and HR is the heart rate (beats/min).

3. $LVSWI = SVI \times (MAP - PAWP) \times 0.0136$ (g-m/m² per beat)

4. $LVSWI = SVI \times (MAP_{SI} - PAWP_{SI}) \times 0.0136 \times 7.5$ (g-m/m² per beat)

where LVSWI is the left ventricle stroke work index, SVI is the stroke volume index (ml/m²), MAP is the mean arterial pressure (mmHg), PAWP is the pulmonary artery wedge pressure (mmHg), MAP_{SI} is the mean arterial pressure (kPa), and $PAWP_{SI}$ is the pulmonary artery wedge pressure (kPa).

5. $RVSWI = SVI \times (MPAP - CVP) \times 0.1036$ (g-m/m² per beat)

6. $RVSWI = SVI \times (MPAP_{SI} - CVP_{SI}) \times 0.1036 \times 7.5$ (g-m/m² per beat)

where RVSWI is the right ventricle stroke work index, SVI is the stroke volume index (ml/m²), MPAP is the mean pulmonary artery pressure (mmHg), CVP is the central venous pressure (mmHg), $MPAP_{SI}$ is the mean pulmonary artery pressure (kPa), and CVP_{SI} is the central venous pressure (kPa).

7. $BSA = 71.84 \times (WT^{0.425}) \times (HT^{0.725})/10\ 000\ (m^2)$

where BSA is the body surface area (DuBois formula), WT is the patient weight (kg) and HT is the patient height (cm).

8. $DO_2 = CaO_2 \times CO \times 10\ (ml\ O_2/min)$

where DO_2 is the oxygen delivery, CaO_2 is the arterial oxygen content (ml/dl) and CO is the cardiac output (liters/min).

9. $CaO_2 = (0.0138 \times HGB \times SaO_2) + (0.0031 \times PaO_2)\ (ml/dl)$

10. $CaO_2 = (0.0138 \times HGB_{SI} \times 1.611 \times SaO_2) + (0.0031 \times PaO_{2SI} \times 7.5)\ (ml/dl)$

where CaO_2 is the arterial oxygen content, HGB is the total hemoglobin (g/dl), SaO_2 is the arterial oxygen saturation (%), PaO_2 is the partial pressure of arterial oxygen (mmHg), HGB_{SI} is the total hemoglobin (mmol/l), and PaO_{2SI} is the partial pressure of arterial oxygen (kPa).

11. $CvO_2 = (0.0138 \times HGB \times SvO_2) + (0.0031 \times PvO_2)\ (ml/dl)$

12. $CvO_2 = (0.0138 \times HGB_{SI} \times 1.611) \times SvO_2) + (0.0031 \times PvO_{2SI} \times 7.5)\ (ml/dl)$

where CvO_2 is the venous oxygen content, HGB is the total hemoglobin (g/dl), SvO_2 is the venous oxygen saturation (%), PvO_2 is the partial pressure of venous oxygen (mmHg), HGB_{SI} is the total hemoglobin (mmol/l), and PvO_{2SI} is the partial pressure of venous oxygen (kPa).

13. $CavO_2 = CaO_2 - CvO_2\ (ml/dl)$

where $CavO_2$ is the arteriovenous oxygen content difference, CaO_2 is the arterial oxygen content (ml/dl) and CvO_2 is the venous oxygen content (ml/dl).

14. $DO_2I = CaO_2 \times CI \times 10\ (ml\ O_2/min\ per\ m^2)$

where DO_2I is the oxygen delivery index, CaO_2 is the arterial oxygen content (ml/dl) and CI is the cardiac index (liters/min per m^2).

$$15.\ VO_2 = CavO_2 \times CO \times 10\ (ml\ O_2/min)$$

where VO_2 is the oxygen consumption, $CavO_2$ is the arteriovenous oxygen content difference (ml/dl) and CO is the cardiac output (liters/min).

$$16.\ VO_2I = CavO_2 \times CI \times 10\ (ml\ O_2/min\ m^2)$$

where VO_2I is the oxygen consumption index, $CavO_2$ is the arteriovenous oxygen content difference (ml/dl), and CI is the cardiac index (liters/min per m^2)

$$17.\ O_2ER = (CavO_2/CaO_2) \times 100\ (\%)$$

where O_2ER is the oxygen extraction ratio, CaO_2 is the arterial oxygen content (ml/dl), $CavO_2$ is the arteriovenous oxygen content difference (ml/dl).

Abbreviations

ABGs	arterial blood gases
ABP	arterial blood pressure
ADH	antidiuretic hormone
ANP	antinatriuretic peptide
APACHE	the Acute Physiology and Chronic Health Evaluation score
ARDS	acute respiratory distress syndrome
ASA	the American Society of Anaesthesiologists physical status scale
ATP	adenosine triphosphate
BSA	body surface area
CaO$_2$	arterial oxygen content
CavO$_2$	arteriovenous oxygen content difference
CCO	continuous cardiac output
CFI	cardiac function index
CI	cardiac index
CO	cardiac output
CvO$_2$	venous oxygen content
CVP	central venous pressure
DO$_2$	oxygen delivery
DO$_2$I	oxygen delivery index
ECG	electrocardiogram
EDV	end-diastolic volume
etCO$_2$	end-tidal carbon dioxide
EVLW	extravascular lung water
FBC	full blood count
FTC	flow time
GCS	Glasgow coma scale
GEDV	global end-diastolic volume
HDU	high dependency unit
HGB	total hemoglobin
HR	heart rate
ICU	intensive care unit
IPPV	intermittent positive pressure ventilation
ITBV	intrathoracic blood volume
LCWI	left cardiac work index

LVEDP	left ventricular end-diastolic pressure
LVEDV	left ventricular end-diastolic volume
LVSWI	left ventricular stroke work index
MAP	mean arterial pressure
MPAP	mean pulmonary artery pressure
NICO	non-invasive cardiac output
O_2ER	oxygen extraction ratio
PaO_2	partial pressure of arterial oxygen
PAWP	pulmonary artery wedge pressure
PCWP	pulmonary capillary wedge pressure
PEEP	positive end-expiratory pressure
P_{IT}	intrathoracic pressure
POSSUM	the Physiological and Operative Severity Score for the Enumeration of Mortality and Morbidity
PPV	pulse pressure variation
P_{TH}	transmural pressure
PvO_2	partial pressure of venous oxygen
PVR	pulmonary vascular resistance
RAP	right arterial pressure
RCWI	right cardiac work index
RVEDV	right ventricular end-diastolic volume
RVSWI	right ventricular stroke work index
S1	first heart sound
S2	second heart sound
SaO_2	arterial oxygen saturation
$ScVO_2$	mixed venous oxygen saturation
SPV	systolic pressure variation
SV	stroke volume
SVI	stroke volume index
SvO_2	venous oxygen saturation
SVR	systemic vascular resistance
SVV	stroke volume variation
TB	blood temperature
TI	injectate temperature
U&Es	urea and electrolytes
VO_2	oxygen consumption
VO_2I	oxygen consumption index

Glossary

Arterial oxygen content (CaO$_2$)
The amount of oxygen carried in the arterial blood, both in the dissolved state and the amount bound to hemoglobin

Arterial oxygen saturation (SaO$_2$)
The percentage of hemoglobin saturated with oxygen in the arterial blood

Arteriovenous oxygen content difference (Ca-vO$_2$)
The difference between the content of oxygen in the arterial and venous side

Autocorrelation
A mathematical method used to derive the length of the heartbeat, overall effect of the heartbeat, or power factor, which is directly in proportion to the nominal, or supposed stroke volume ejected from the aorta

Baseline blood temperature
Blood temperature that serves as the basis for cardiac output measurements

Blood temperature (BT)
The temperature of the blood in the pulmonary artery when the catheter is properly positioned

Body surface area (BSA)
The surface area of a patient's skin

Bolus injection
A known volume of iced or room-temperature fluid, which is injected into a port on the pulmonary artery catheter and serves as the indicator for measuring cardiac output

Cardiac function index (CFI)
Reflects cardiac contractile function

Cardiac index (CI)
Cardiac output adjusted for body size

Cardiac output (CO)
The volume of blood ejected per minute from the heart into the systemic circulation

Central venous pressure (CVP)
The mean pressure in the superior vena cava (right atrium); it indicates venous return to the right side of the heart

Computation constant
A constant used in the cardiac output equation that accounts for the density of blood in an injectate, the injectate volume and the indicator loss in the catheter

Continuous mode
The functional state in which cardiac output is trended on a continuous basis

Ejection fraction
The percentage of the end-diastolic volume represented by the stroke volume

End-diastolic volume (EDV)
The amount of blood in each ventricle at the end of ventricular diastole (or start of systole)

End-diastolic volume index (EDVI)
The right heart end-diastolic volume adjusted for body size

End-systolic volume (ESV)
The amount of blood remaining in each ventricle at the end of ventricular systole (the start of ventricular diastole)

End-systolic volume index (ESVI)
The right heart end-systolic volume adjusted for body size

End-tidal carbon dioxide (etCO$_2$)
The carbon dioxide content of an exhaled volume

Extravascular lung water (EVLW)
Reflects the level of pulmonary edema, if increased

Fraction of inspired oxygen (FiO$_2$)
The fraction of oxygen in the inspired air

Heart rate (HR)
The number of ventricular contractions per minute

Hemoglobin (HGB)
The oxygen-carrying component of the red blood cells

Indicator
A dye, fluid (room-temperature or ice-cold), drug or heat filament that can be detected by introducing it into the cardiovascular system and detecting it at another point downstream

Injectate
The fluid used for bolus thermodilution cardiac output measurement

Injectate temperature (IT)
The measured temperature of the injectate used for bolus thermodilution cardiac output measurement

Intrathoracic blood volume (ITBV)
A volumetric measure of cardiac preload

Left ventricular stroke work index (LVSWI)
A measure of the amount of work the left ventricle exerts during systole, adjusted for body size

Mean arterial pressure (MAP)
The average systemic arterial blood pressure

Mean pulmonary artery pressure (MPAP)
The average blood pressure measured in the pulmonary artery

Mixed venous oxygen saturation (ScVO$_2$)
The percentage of hemoglobin saturated with oxygen in the venous blood as measured in the pulmonary artery

Oxygen consumption (VO$_2$)
The amount of oxygen used by the tissues

Oxygen consumption index (VO$_2$I)
The amount of oxygen used by the tissues, adjusted for body size

Oxygen delivery (DO$_2$)
The amount of oxygen delivered to the tissues

Oxygen delivery index (DO$_2$I)
The amount of oxygen delivered to the tissues, adjusted for body size

Oxygen extraction index (O$_2$EI)
This is determined by using dual oximetry, SaO$_2$ and SvO$_2$, and evaluates the ratio of oxygen extracted to the amount of oxygen supplied

Oxygen extraction ratio (O$_2$ER)
This is the ratio of oxygen content difference to the amount of oxygen supplied

Pulmonary capillary wedge pressure (PCWP)
The pressure obtained from the pulmonary artery catheter when the balloon is inflated and the catheter tip progresses into a more distal branch of the pulmonary artery. It reflects left atrial pressure in the absence of mechanical obstruction between the balloon tip and the left atrium

Pulmonary vascular resistance (PVR)
A derived measure of impedance to blood flow from right ventricle (afterload)

Pulmonary vascular resistance index (PVRI)
Pulmonary vascular resistance adjusted for body size

Pulse contour
Analysis of the shape/systolic part of the arterial waveform in order to derive a nominal stroke volume

Pulse power
Analysis of the power of the whole arterial waveform in order to derive a nominal stroke volume

Right ventricular stroke work index (RVSWI)
A measure of the amount of work the right ventricle exerts during systole, adjusted for body size

Signal
The induced temperature change that is used to measure cardiac output

Stroke volume (SV)
The amount of blood pumped out of each ventricle during a single beat

Stroke volume index (SVI)
Stroke volume adjusted for body size

Stroke volume variation (SVV)
A continuous indicator of volume responsiveness (only in patients on fully controlled mechanical ventilation)

Systemic vascular resistance (SVR)
A derived measure of impedance to blood flow from left ventricle (afterload)

Systemic vascular resistance index (SVRI)
Systemic vascular resistance adjusted for body size

Thermal filament
The area on the continuous cardiac output thermodilution catheter that transfers small amounts of energy into the blood to serve as indicator for trending cardiac output continuously

Thermistor
A temperature sensor near the tip of the pulmonary artery catheter

Thermodilution
A variant of the indicator dilution technique using temperature change as the indicator

Transducer
A fluid-filled system that senses and converts a signal into a digital value and/or waveform on to a monitor/amplifier

Transpulmonary
The cold bolus traverses the lungs after being injected through a CVP line and the thermodilution curve is being measured in a systemic artery

Trend
A collection of historical data points

Venous oxygen content (CvO_2)
The amount of oxygen carried in the venous blood, both in the dissolved state and the amount bound to hemoglobin

Venous oxygen saturation (SvO_2)
The percentage of hemoglobin saturated with oxygen in the venous blood

Ventilation perfusion index (VQI)
This is determined by using dual oximetry, SaO_2 and SvO_2. This value is a derivation of the intrapulmonary shunt equation and provides an estimate of intrapulmonary shunt value

Washout curve
An indicator dilution curve produced by a bolus injection. Cardiac output is inversely related to the area under this curve

Waveform
The graphical representation of digital values (e.g. pressure, flow, impedance, volume) obtained from a sensed signal

Bibliography

Ahrens T, Rutherford K 1993 Essentials of oxygenation. Mass Jones & Bartlett, Boston

Albin G, Rahko P S 1990 Comparison of echocardiographic quantitation of left-ventricular ejection fraction to radionuclide angiography in patients with regional wall motion abnormalities. American Journal of Cardiology 65: 1031–1032

Anonymous 1998 Annual report from the national case mix programme database. Intensive Care National Audit and Research Centre, London

Appel S, Kram H 1998 Oxygen transport measurements to evaluate tissue perfusion and titrate therapy: dobutamine and dopamine effects. Critical Care Medicine 19: 672–687

Audit Commission 1995 United they stand. Co-ordinating care for elderly patients with hip fracture. HMSO Publications, London

Babu S C, Sharma P V P, Raciti A et al 1980 Monitor-guided responses – operability with safety is increased in patients with peripheral vascular disease. Archives of Surgery 115: 1384

Band D M, Linton R A F, Jonas M M, Linton N W F 1997 The shape of indicator dilution curves used for cardiac output measurements in man. Journal of Physiology 498: 225–229

Barone J E, Snyder A B 1991 Treatment strategies in shock: use of oxygen transport measurements. Heart and Lung 20: 81–85

Bashein G, Johnson P W, Davis K B, Ivey T D 1985 Elective coronary bypass surgery without pulmonary artery catheter monitoring. Anesthesiology 63: 451

Beique F A, Lavoie J 1998 TEE monitoring. Canadian Journal of Anaesthaesia 45(10): 919–924

Berlauk J F, Abrams J H, Gilmour I J, O'Connor S R, Knighton D R, Cerra F B 1991 Preoperative optimisation of cardiovascular hemodynamics improves outcome in peripheral vascular surgery: a prospective, randomised clinical trial. Annals of Surgery 214: 289–299

Berwick D M, Leape L L. Reducing errors in medicine. British Medical Journal 319: 136–137

Bland M J, Altman D J 1986 Statistical methods for assessing agreement between two methods of clinical measurement. Lancet 1: 3071986 310

Boyd O 2003 Optimisation of oxygenation and tissue perfusion in surgical patients. Intensive and Critical Care Nursing 19: 171–181

Burchell S A, Yu M, Edwards J D 1997 Invasive techniques for the estimation of cardiac output. International Journal of Intensive Care Summer: 44–50

Burchell S A, Yu M, Takiguchi S A, Ohta R M, Myers S A 1997 Evaluation of a continuous cardiac output and mixed venous oxygen saturation catheter in critically ill surgical patients. Critical Care Medicine 25, 3: 388–391

Cariou A, Monchi M, Joly L M et al 1998 Noninvasive cardiac output monitoring by aortic blood flow determination: evaluation of the Sometec Dynemo-3000 system. Critical Care Medicine 26: 2066–2072

Chaney J C, Derdak S 2002 Minimally invasive hemodynamic monitoring for the intensivist: current and emerging technology. Critical Care Medicine 30: 2338–2345

Cheung A T, Savino J S, Weiss S J, Aukburg S J, Berlin J A 1994 Echocardiographic and hemodynamic indexes of left ventricular preload in patients with normal and abnormal ventricular function. Anesthesiology 81: 376–387

Cholley B P, Shroff S G, Sandelski J et al 1995 Differential effects of chronic oral antihypertensive therapies on systemic arterial circulation and ventricular energetics in African–American patients. Circulation 91: 1052–1062

Copel L C, Stolarik A 1991 Continuous SAO_2 monitoring: a research review. Dimensions of Critical Care Nursing 10: 202–209

Del Guercio L R M, Cohn J D 1980 Monitoring operative risk in the elderly. JAMA 243: 1350

Dubois R W, Brook R H 1988 Preventable deaths: who, how often and why? Annals of International Medicine 109: 582–589

Esperson K, Jensen E W, Rosenborg D, Thomsen J K, Eliasen K, Olsen N V, Kanstrup I L 1995 Comparison of cardiac output measurement techniques: thermodilution, Doppler, CO_2 rebreathing and the direct Fick method. Acta Anaesthesiologica Scandinavica 39: 245–511

Forrester J S, Ganz W, Diamond G, McHugh T, Chonette D W, Swan H J C 1972 Thermodilution cardiac output determination with a single flow-directed catheter. American Heart Journal 83: 306–311

Gattinoni L, Brazzi L, Pelosi P et al 1995 A trial of goal-oriented hemodynamic therapy in critically ill patients, SvO_2 Collaborative Group. New England Journal of Medicine 333: 1025

Gedeon A, Forslund L, Hedenstierna G, Romano E 1980 A new method for noninvasive bedside determination of pulmonary blood flow. Medical and Biological Engineering and Computing 18: 411–418

George A, Folk B P, Crecelius P L, Cambell W B 1989 Pre-arrest morbidity and other correlates of survival after in-hospital cardiopulmonary arrest. American Journal of Medicine 87: 28–34

Goedje O, Hoeke K, Lichtwarck-Aschoff M et al 1999 Continuous cardiac output by femoral arterial thermodilution calibrated pulse contour analysis: comparison with pulmonary arterial thermodilution. Critical Care Medicine 27: 2407–2412

Gregory I C 1974 The oxygen and carbon monoxide capacities of foetal and adult blood. Journal of Physiology 236: 625

Gunn S R, Pinsky M R 2001 Implications of arterial pressure variation in patients in the intensive care unit. Current Opinion in Critical Care 7: 212–217

Gutierrez G, Wulf M 1996 Lactic acidosis in sepsis: a commentary. Intensive Care Medicine 22: 6–16

Headley J 1995 Strategies to optimize the cardiorespiratory status of the critically ill. American Association of Critical Care Clinical Issues 6(1): 121–134

Jacobsen C J 1995 Invasive cardiac output monitoring. Costs, complications and benefits of new systems. International Journal of Intensive Care Summer: 1995

Kaplan A 2002 The potential to replace more invasive monitoring techniques [letter]. Critical Care Medicine 30(8): 1933

Kelman G R 1966 Digital computer subroutine for the conversion of oxygen tension into saturation. Journal of Applied Physiology 21: 1375–1376

Kelman G R, Nunn J F 1966 Nomograms for correction of blood pO_2, pCO_2, pH and base excess for time and temperature. Journal of Applied Physiology 21: 1484–1490

Kern J W, Shoemaker W C 2002 Meta-analysis of hemodynamic optimisation in high-risk patients. Critical Care Medicine 30(8): 1686–1692

Lawrence A, Havill J H 1999 An audit of deaths occurring in hospital after discharge from intensive care unit. Anesthesia Intensive Care 27: 185–189

Linton R A, Young L E, Marlin D J et al 2000 Cardiac output measured by lithium dilution, thermodilution and transesophageal Doppler echocardiography in anesthetized horses. American Journal of Veterinary Research 61(7): 7317

Loeb R G, Brown E A, DiNardo J A, Orr J A, Watt R C 1999 Clinical accuracy of a new non-invasive cardiac output monitor. Anesthesiology V91(3A): A474

McGloin H, Adam S K, Singer M 1999 Unexpected deaths and referrals to intensive care of patient on general wards. Are some cases potentially avoidable? Journal of the Royal College of Physicians 33: 255–259

McQuillan P, Pilkington S, Allan A et al 1998 Confidential inquiry into quality of care before admission to intensive care. British Medical Journal 316: 1853–1858

Mitchell J P, Schuller D, Calandrin F S, Schuster D 1992 Improved outcome based on fluid management in critically ill patients requiring pulmonary artery catheterisation. American Review of Respiratory Diseases 145: 990–998

Model SAT-2 Oximeter/cardiac output operations manual [computer program] 1991 Software version 7.12. Baxter Healthcare Corporation, Irvine, CA

Monchi M, Thebert D, Cariou A et al 1998 Clinical evaluation of the Abbott Qvue-OptiQ continuous cardiac output system in critically ill medical patients. Journal of Critical Care 13: 91–95

Moore C H, Lombardo T R, Allums J A, Gordon F T 1978 Left main coronary artery stenosis: hemodynamic monitoring to reduce mortality. Annals of Thoracic Surgery 26: 445

Munro B H, Visintainer M A, Page E B 1986 Statistical methods for health care research. JB Lippincott Co., Philadelphia

Mythen M G, Webb A R 1994 Intra-operative gut mucosal hypoperfusion is associated with increased post-operative complications and cost. Intensive Care Medicine 20: 99–104

Mythen M G, Webb A R 1995 Perioperative plasma volume expansion reduces the incidence of gut mucosal hypoperfusion during cardiac surgery. Archives of Surgery 130: 423–429

Neale G 1998 Risk management in the care of medical emergencies after referral to hospital. Journal of the Royal College of Physicians 32: 125–129

Nethirasigamani D, Fielden J M 2002 Pre-operative optimisation of high risk surgical patients [letter]. Anaesthesia 57: 405–406

Nightingale P 1990 Practical points in the application of oxygen transport principles. Intensive Care Medicine 16: S173–S177

Poelart J, Schmidt C, Van Aken H, Hinder F, Molhoff T, Loick M A 1999 Comparison of transoesophageal echocardiographic Doppler across the aortic valve and thermodilution technique per estimating cardiac output. Anaesthesia 54: 128

Poeze M, Greve J W, Ramsay G 2000 Goal-oriented haemodynamic therapy: a plea for a closer look at using perioperative oxygen transport. Intensive Care Medicine 26: 635–637

Pond C, Blessions G, Bowlin J, McCawley C, Lappas D 1992 Perioperative evaluation of a new mixed venous oxygen saturation catheter in cardiac surgical patients. Journal of Cardiovascular Vascular Anesthesia 3: 280–282

Reinersten J L 2000 Let's talk about error. British Medical Journal 320: 730

Resuscitation Council [UK] 2000 ALS manual, 4th edn. Resuscitation Council, London

Reuter D, Felbinger T, Kilger E et al 2001 Optimising fluid therapy in mechanically ventilated patients after cardiac surgery by on-line monitoring of left ventricular stroke volume variations. Comparison with aortic systolic pressure variations. British Journal of Anaesthesia 88: 124–126

Sakka S G, Reinhart K, Meier-Hellmann A 1999 Comparison of pulmonary artery and arterial thermodilution cardiac output in critically ill patients. Intensive Care Medicine 25: 843–846

Sakka S G, Meier Hellmann A, Reinhart K 2000 Assessment of intrathoracic blood volume and extravascular lung water by single transpulmonary thermodilution. Intensive Care Medicine 26: 180–187

Savino J S, Hanson C W III, Bigelow D C, Cheung A T, Weiss S J 1994 Oropharyngeal injury after transesophageal echocardiography. Journal Cardiothoracic and Vascular Anesthesia 8: 76–78

Schein R M, Hazday N, Pena M, Ruben B H, Sprung C L 1990 Clinical antecedents to in-hospital cardiopulmonary arrest. Chest 98: 1388–1392

Scuderi P E, MacGregor D A, Bowton D L, James R L 1994 A laboratory comparison of three pulmonary artery oximetry catheters. Anesthesiology 81: 245–253

Shoemaker W C, Kram H B, Appel P L, Fleming A W 1990 The efficacy of central venous and pulmonary artery catheters and therapy based upon them in reducing mortality and morbidity. Archives of Surgery 125: 1332–1338

Shoemaker W C, Thangathurai D, Wo C C et al 1999 Intraoperative evaluation of tissue perfusion in high-risk patients by invasive and non-invasive hemodynamic monitoring. Critical Care Medicine 27(10): 2147–2152

Side C D, Gosling R J 1971 Non-surgical assessment of cardiac function. Nature 232: 335–336

Silance P G, Simon C, Vincent J L 1994 The relation between cardiac index and oxygen extraction in acutely ill patients. Chest 105: 1190–1197

Singh S, Manji M 2001 A survey of pre-operative optimisation of high-risk surgical patients undergoing major elective surgery. Anaesthesia 56: 988–1002

Smith A F, Wood J 1998 Can some in-hospital cardio-pulmonary arrests be prevented? A prospective study. Resuscitation 37: 133–127

Smith G B, Nielsen M S 1998 Criteria for admission. British Medical Journal 318: 1544–1547

Stamm R B, Carabello B A, Mayers D L et al 1982 Two dimensional echocardiographic measurement of left-ventricular ejection fraction: prospective analysis of what

constitutes an adequate determination. American Heart
Journal 104: 136–144

Teboul J, Graini L, Boujdaria R, Berton C, Richard C 1993
Cardiac index vs oxygen-derived parameters for rational use
of dobutamine in patients with congestive heart failure. Chest
103: 81–85

Thomas L J 1972 Algorithms for selected blood acid-base and
blood gas calculations. Journal of Applied Physiology 33:
154–158

Trunet P, Le Gall J-R, Lhoste F et al 1980 The role of iatrogenic
disease in admissions to intensive care. JAMA 244:
2617–2620

Ultman J S, Bursztein S 1981 Analysis of error in the
determination of respiratory gas exchange at varying FIO_2.
Journal of Applied Physiology 50: 210–216

Vallet B, Lebuffe G, Wiel E 2003 High risk surgical patients: why
should we optimise? In: Yearbook of intensive care and
emergency medicine. Springer, Heidelberg: 57–67

Van der Hoeven J G 1999 Intensive care medicine in the next
millennium: exciting developments versus cost containment.
Netherlands Journal of Medicine 55: 297–299

Van der Hoeven, JG, Olsman J 1999 Preoptimisation of oxygen
delivery – intensive care moves into preventative care.
Netherlands Journal of Medicine 54: 213–214

Watt R C, Loeb R G, Orr J 1998 Comparison of a new non-
invasive cardiac output technique with invasive bolus and
continuous thermodilution. Anesthesiology 89(3a): A536

West J B, Dollery C T, Naimark A 1964 Distribution of blood
flow in isolated lung: relation to vascular and alveolar
pressures. Journal of Applied Physiology 19: 713

Wilson R J, Woods I 2001 Cardiovascular optimisation for high-
risk surgery. Current Opinions in Crititical Care 7: 195–199

Wolfe R 1992 Glucose metabolism. In: Wolfe R (ed.)
Radioactive and stable isotope tracers in biomedicine:
principles and practice of kinetic analysis. Wiley-Liss, New
York, 283–315

Yu M, Levy M M, Smith P, Takiguchi S A, Miyasaki A, Myers S A
1993 Effect of maximum oxygen delivery on mobility and
mortality in critically ill patients: a prospective, randomised
controlled study. Critical Care Medicine 21: 830–838

Index